Lucille D. Catalano

Martinis
and
Whipped Cream

Sidney Petrie
in association with **Robert B. Stone**

Martinis
and
Whipped Cream

The New *Carbo-Cal* Way
to Lose Weight
and Stay Slim

Parker Publishing Company, West Nyack, N. Y.

Lovingly Dedicated
to
Fannie and Jack

A Doctor's Foreword to This Book

Physicians have known the truth about carbohydrates in weight control for decades. It is their patients who have either never been able to understand it or who have not applied their knowledge of it to their daily eating habits.

The basic truth is—we eat too much of carbohydrates. If we ate less of them we'd be much healthier. Eating excessively of carbohydrates is the prime cause of excessive poundage. As a family physician I see this demonstrated every day, and I do put the finger of blame on lack of dietary education.

We physicians also know that carbohydrates fatten you more easily than other types of foods. Suppose you ate nothing but apple pie all day. One serving for breakfast, one for lunch, one for dinner and another thrown in for good measure. Would these be filling meals? Not in the least. You would be hungry even though this would be equivalent to approximately 1600 calories. Apple pie is almost 100% carbohydrate. You might also gain weight. On the other hand, just for comparison, if you had four meals consisting of two strips of bacon and two eggs each, you would be eating less than 1000 calories and thus, probably would lose weight because this type of meal is 100% free of carbohydrate. Furthermore, you'd have that "full" feeling for a longer period of time.

I am not suggesting that you cut down your carbohydrate intake to zero. The body needs a certain amount of carbohydrates to properly assimilate and metabolize the proteins and fats. If you gave it none, it might borrow from its own carbohydrate storeroom for a while, but then health troubles would arise. The exact amount of carbohydrate that is needed for any given indi-

vidual is presently unknown. Fifty grams of carbohydrate a day
might be called a safe minimum for most people. That equals
about 200 calories a day. The authors ask you to keep your
carbohydrate calorie intake down to 250 a day. This certainly
leaves a margin of safety, albeit a narrow range.

By learning how to cut down on carbohydrates in this book
you really are not going on a "diet." It can be possible to eat
more and shed pounds. There is nothing *off* your list. You will
be learning how to eat what you should eat. You will enjoy food
more and live longer to enjoy food.

MILTON C. KEMP, M.D.

What This Book Will Do for You

Dieting to lose weight can now be a thing of the past. The gnawing hunger, the war with one's self, the celery stalks, the broken promises—all may soon be forgotten. Gone, too, will be the slow but sure regaining of the pounds and the need to start the torture all over again!

Instead, we are entering a new era of eat well, drink well, and weigh less; an era when martinis, filet mignon and whipped cream replace the skimmed milk, carrot sticks and melba toast of that on-again, off-again diet age.

The carbohydrate calorie is more fattening than any other kind of calorie. This is the scientific fact that is now revolutionizing the eating habits of millions. By using this fact in their daily lives, people are now literally able to eat more and weigh less! Slender people can enjoy a hearty breakfast, a mid-morning coffee break, a "Madison Avenue lunch," an afternoon cocktail hour, a gourmet dinner, and a midnight snack—and still remain slender.

No longer does one need to count every calorie consumed, or to measure portions ounce by ounce. *Only the villain carbohydrates need be watched.* We do not have to watch our step on proteins, or even fats. Eliminate as much carbohydrate as we can and fat melts away. Enjoy the double-size vodka martinis, bigger portions of roast beef, and "seconds" on strawberries and cream, and still lose weight.

What is more—you can kiss that lost weight goodbye *forever.* This is true for the simple reason that you are not on a restrictive regime by dint of willpower or resolve. There is really no diet to slip from. The only thing you can do to gain back those life-shortening pounds is to give up your caviar and eggs benedict and decide to go back to a life of spaghetti, bread and potatoes.

People today are more weight-conscious than ever before. We know the penalty of excess poundage in illness, lessened energy, lower life expectancy, and general unattractiveness. We have dieted and dieted and *dieted.* We have become ashamed of ourselves as each spell of dieting ended and our weight gradually returned. We blamed our weak willpower and our weaker character, when actually the blame has rested the whole while on the creeping encroachment of carbohydrates into our modern foods.

Now all that is over. Happy eating and drinking days are here again! It is no longer true that good things in life are either illegal or fattening. We may not be able to have our cake and be slender too. But we can eat and drink as we never have before, and keep slim and trim. And this book will show just how it can work for you.

Contents

CONTENTS

1

You Can
Eat More . . .

Anybody can lose weight—just stop eating. This is obviously impossible for the average person, so hardly anybody loses weight. If we do manage to lose weight by cutting down on eating, we gain it right back when we start eating regularly again.

Suppose the truth were: Anybody can lose weight—just eat more. Then everybody would lose weight. This would indeed be a country of slender, healthy attractive people with a life expectancy of years more.

. . . And Weigh Less

The fact is: *You can eat more and weigh less!*

Much is now being said and written about the low carbohydrate diet. Hundreds of thousands of people are now trying it. Many are literally eating better than they ever have before and watching the pounds melt away. They are drinking martinis, washing their Long Island duckling down with goblets of red wine, living it up with strawberries and whipped cream and literally having

1

an epicurean ball while their on-the-wagon, cottage cheese and carrot stick friends wonder how they do it.

Has the calorie been wrongly accused, and has the carbohydrate been the villain right along? *Yes* and *no*. Calories do count, but carbohydrate calories count more than any others. Carbohydrate calories add weight faster than protein or fat calories.

If you are slowly and steadily gaining weight now, by using the information in this book you can eat as much as you are eating now and be slowly and steadily losing weight. Since you are not cutting down on food, there is hardly any willpower involved. No hunger. No irritability. No monotony. No body-less, taste-less, flavor-less foods. There is no diet to end. You are merely substituting one kind of food for another. So there is no sad ending, no gaining back of lost weight.

This may sound like a happy book. It is! For overweight people, or for those who just want to make it into a size 12, this is probably the happiest book ever. It shows you how you can eat as much and as often as you want, enjoy those two martinis (or three) before dinner, and that brandy after dinner, and still keep your weight in check.

The Eating Man's Diet

A stenographer, 37 years of age, had been on and off a dozen diets in as many years, and was now at 166 pounds, the most she had ever weighed. In the first week she lost seven pounds. In one month she lost 18 pounds, in two months 27 pounds. How long did she diet and how much did she lose? Here's what she has to say a year later: "I am off carbohydrates for good. I enjoy this new way of eating. I weigh 128. I feel that both my weight and hunger problems are over."

Some cases are really dramatic. One young man weighed 280 pounds. Every time he tried to diet he gave it up in a short time and indulged himself back to an even higher weight than when he started. The low carbohydrate diet was made to order for him.

He had a big appetite. He switched from dry cereals for breakfast to eggs and ham, bacon or sausage—not just one egg and one slice of bacon, but three and four eggs if he felt like it—and as much bacon as his appetite demanded. (This was usually closer to eight slices.) Similarly, lunch and dinner were hearty meals. His weight literally dove down and kept diving. In seven months he was down 90 pounds and not a hunger pang along the way!

In the past ten years the author has seen this success story repeated in different ways for a thousand people. In just about every case, there was no hunger, no regaining of lost weight. He has watched progress chart after progress chart develop its inevitable downward curve with only an occasional leveling off between dips. Close observation by physicians and family doctors found no ill effects. In fact, many difficulties being treated lessened or disappeared with the increased vitality that weight loss brought.

This book teaches you how to recognize high carbohydrate foods and how to limit your intake of these weight hooks. A plate of spaghetti can, under certain circumstances, be the hook for a pound of fat to hang itself to you. But a two pound steak can go through you and leave only a trace of bone and muscle mending protein once its energy has been consumed. It helps you understand how modern living came to be over-saturated with these fattening-carbohydrates and how giving them up for heartier foods can add years to your life. It provides you with carbohydrate tables for every food you have ever heard of, and many you haven't. It gives you simple charts of "go" foods, "caution" foods, and "stop" foods, based not on calorie value (these are listed, too) but on carbohydrate content.

This book also helps you transfer your kitchen shelves from human fat larders to storehouses of body-building protein. It removes taboos and shows you how to enjoy healthful foods. It gives you a green light on celebrating and party-hopping and arms you with the information you need to enjoy yourself without conscience pangs. It gives you recipes, menus, and gourmet cooking tips. And it backs it all up with scientific fact, medical endorsement, and case histories totaling thousands upon thousands of lost pounds.

The Melba Toast Myth

When you count calories and ignore what kind of calories you count, you find that carrot sticks and melba toast are fine. But if you count *carbohydrate* calories, you find that carrots have two and three times more fat producer than such nutritious vegetables as squash, string beans, cabbage, turnips, cauliflower, mushrooms, asparagus and many more; while melba toast and zweiback are higher in fattening carbohydrate calories than double their weight in any other bread or toast you can mention.

Turning a friendly eye on low carbohydrate content turns up such welcome foods as cheese—Cheddar, Limburger, Liederkranz, Camembert, Roquefort, Gorgonzola, and many more including cream cheese; meat—steaks, roast beef, lamb, pork, veal, sausage, frankfurters, hamburgers; poultry and game—chicken, turkey, duck, goose, squab, rabbit; fish—just about any fish and saltwater fish or shellfish you can think of, cooked any way you like, even fried (but not breaded); and scores of fruits, vegetables, eggs and dairy products.

In addition—sauces, gravies, and dressings formerly taboo by calorie counting standards became very much permissible by carbohydrate standards. Say "hello" to hollandaise and butter sauces; to natural juice and fat gravies; to mayonnaise, oils and tartar sauce. If you like to cook with wine, be happy, the world of dry wines is yours.

Most people who enjoy drinking have had that enjoyment blunted by the thought that liquor is fattening. There is not a trace of fattening carbohydrates in gin and vodka; nor is there any in scotch, bourbon and rye wiskey; or in rum and most brandies. Only beer drinkers will have to count, and only cordial and liqueur drinkers will have to switch. For the cocktail hour or two, sip away to your heart's content on Manhattans, dry Martinis and Bacardis.

Many surprises are in store for you when you gauge fattening foods by the more efficient carbohydrate measuring stick. Custard is far less fattening than jello. Vanilla ice cream is lower on the carbohydrate percentage table than lemon ice or milk sherbert. Whipped cream is only 1.1% carbohydrate, buttermilk is 4.6%, skimmed milk is 5%. But we are getting ahead of ourselves.

What Is the Low-Carbohydrate Way?

Compared to diets, the low carbohydrate way is permissive rather than restrictive. It is therefore somewhat unfair to call it a diet, but more recently it has been referred to as the drinking man's diet, the Air Force diet, and the low carbohydrate diet. The author prefers to call it the low carbohydrate way of losing or maintaining weight.

If you don't count calories—what do you do? You eat and drink all you want of low carbohydrate foods called "go" foods in the chapters ahead. You count only when you eat some medium or high carbohydrate foods called "caution" and "stop" foods. For these you count only their carbohydrate calories.

If you stay on "go" foods, you have no counting at all to do. You can go days without so much as a pause to wonder or figure. If you decide you want some of the higher carbohydrate foods, go right ahead. But check the simple tables provided later in the book to determine what carbohydrate calories to charge against your daily limit. Because the carbohydrate calorie has a different effect on the body than other food calories, it needs a name to set it apart. "Carbo-cal" seems a natural. You will be using that word constantly from now on as you enjoy eating all you want—thanks to the fact that you limit your Carbo-cals.

This carbohydrate limit is set by you. You decide what your daily carbohydrate ceiling should be, according to whether you want to lose weight fast or gradually, or whether you just want to maintain your present slim figure. This limit can allow you a daily sandwich or dessert. It permits an occasional coke or a spaghetti dinner. But this is where the serious counting begins and where some of the sweet foods end. Let's not fool ourselves. Carbohydrates turn to fat and fat is a killer.

Our Modern Carbohydrate Way of Life

Modern technology has made its mark on the food industry. Prepared foods have emancipated the housewife—given her more free time. And there is more of her to enjoy that time. She weighs more, her husband weighs more, and the children are chubbier. Carbohydrates lend themselves to all manner of "goodies." What used to be a rare treat that grandmother would surprise us with is now piled six feet high on the supermarket cookie shelves in more sizes, shapes and flavors than you can count. The only surprise comes if you open the shopping bags at home and find that you forgot them.

Remember the rolling pin? It used to be one of mother's most useful kitchen utensils, flattening out dough for noodles, pie crusts and tarts. Baking these treats was an all-day proposition and many a hand got slapped reaching for one before it was cool or before the proper occasion for eating.

Today, spaghetti and noodles are assembly line products; breads, rolls, doughnuts, pastries and cakes are baked in factories and delivered by fleets of trucks; and new products like pizzas, ice cream and potato chips join the fattening parade.

What happened to grandmother? She's now only a few steps from the kitchen, watching television, listening to the radio or reading the newspapers, and deciding which frozen pie to buy or which cold cereal to try next. And even if such decisions couldn't be further from her mind, she, mother, and the rest of the family are still being exposed to the constant barrage of appetizing sales talks that proclaim one carbohydrate-packed product to be better than the other.

There are no lamb chop commercials, no roast turkey or broiled sword fish sales pitches. Not even a mention of martinis or whipped cream. But our vast subconscious storehouse of motivating impulses is charged again and again with the easiness of cake and pancake mixes, the deliciousness of ready made buns and rolls, and the common-sense practicality of the large double pack of crackers. Little wonder when we roll that cart down the market aisle, we fill it three-quarters full of carbo-cals.

If we are health-conscious, our reason is appeased by statements on the packages that the pop-in-the-toaster waffles contain all the daily requirements of riboflavin or other vitamins and that this brand of spaghetti is highest in protein. (In reality, as high as a sand dune in a desert of carbohydrate.) We are impressed also by the healthy-looking specimens of humanity that quaff down more than one beer with that brewed-in flavor.

The fact is, the carbo-cal kills more people each year than cancer, war and the automobile combined. The first 300 to 500 carbo-cals you consume each day are nice to you. They take their place in the energy-producing furnace of your body and literally go to work for you. Any additional carbo-cals after that take their place on your waist line, buttocks, thighs, arms and wherever else they can squeeze in, *and you go to work for them.* You heat them, nourish them and transport them. The thanks you get is shapelessness and unattractiveness, rising weight and falling level of health.

A Low-Carbohydrate Diet Is a Balanced Diet

It is a fact of life to nutritionists and dieticians that Americans consume too much sugar and carbohydrate. The volume of suggestions that you are bombarded with hourly by radio and TV commercials, advertisements, billboards and see-through packages has affected your eating habits. It pays to advertise, and, certainly where carbohydrates are concerned, *you* have been paying.

Cutting back on carbo-cals, therefore, does not unbalance your diet. In fact, it restores its balance. Reducing carbo-cal intake to 20% or 25% of your total returns your way of eating closer to the natural balance that existed before mass distribtuion methods upset it. The recent revived interest in low carbohydrate diets has been accompanied by dire warnings of the need for this food in the body's proper functioning. This is absolutely true. Carbohydrates are essential. They must be a part of daily food consumption. Nothing in this category should be completely eliminated. To reduce carbohydrate intake to below the recommended minimums would be like taking an overdose of medicine.

Looking at the positive aspect of this, you should not feel guilty when you dig in to the dish of ice cream or enjoy that danish pastry with your coffee. True, it is a once-a-day affair—thus far and no further. But, within such limits, it is good for you. *Bon appetit!*

Part of the advantage of reading this book from cover to cover will be its help to you in counteracting the pro-carbohydrate conditioning that reaches you each day. This book will, in effect, provide equal time for the chopped tenderloin steak smothered in mushrooms. When you are not watching television commercials, these pages will bombard you with ideas for tempting snacks, gourmet recipes for savoury casseroles, and exciting menus with an international flavor—all part of a balanced and nourishing daily fare as far removed from the diet concept as you can get.

The ads for cereals and cinnamon buns do not mention these foods as part of a regimented diet upon which you should embark. Yet the very fact that someone comes into your living room a score or more times a day to entice you with rhythm and catchy slogan to buy and eat these foods (always held on camera for you to see), influences you to give these foods a larger and larger place in your daily living. They become a diet. Over the years you have actually gone on a diet of carbo-cals with a minimum of daily protein. It is *out of balance* and contrary to good health.

If you are now reminded in an equally convincing way of gustatory delights of protein, and you respond by revising your shopping list, there can come about, without any mention of diet, a new balanced way of eating. Optimistically, you will be going on a diet of fats and proteins with closer to a minimum of daily carbo-cals. It is *in balance* and conducive to good health.

The Low Cost of Proteins Versus Carbohydrates

There is no doubt that two pounds of sirloin steak are more expensive than two pounds of macaroni. Bread and potatoes fill up the shopping bags and later the dinner plates, for only nickels, while the ingredients for a chef's salad with roquefort cream dressing add up to dimes and maybe quarters. On the surface carbohydrates appear to be a less expensive way to eat, and, after all, budgets must be kept within bounds.

But when you look beneath the surface, as a budget-conscious shopper you get some second thoughts. Have you ever heard someone complain how, after a huge Chinese dinner, they are soon hungry again? The rice, oriental noodles and corn starch cookery is high in carbo-cals, low in lasting value. The same is true of our corn flake breakfasts and sandwich and malted lunches. The breakfast is soon followed by a second breakfast (make it Danish, so it won't spoil your appetite for lunch), and the sandwich lunch is often followed by a cake-and-coffee afternoon break that seldom affects your appetite for dinner.

When it comes to supplying fuel to your house you measure the initial cost against the lasting power of the fuel. When it comes to supplying fuel to your body, you measure the initial cost alone, and let it go at that. Carbohydrates are cheaper, yes. But, in the long run you get much more mileage from your protein dollar.

Carrying the analogy one step further—when buying fuel or lubricant for your car, you would avoid like the plague any cheaper and inferior product that you fear might cause excessive wear or damage to the motor. There you are not penny-wise and pound-foolish, to use an old British monetary expression. Why not then avoid like the plague (which they are) those cheaper, inferior carbo-cals that add excessive weight and damage your body? This might not be penny-wise, but it is very pound-foolish, using "pound" in its weighty sense.

Over the long run, carbo-cals are more expensive. One dollar a day of excessive carbo-cal intake may reduce a man's earning power by a hundred thousand dollars in his lifetime. Increase the cost of a breakfast by 30 cents worth of bacon and eggs and you save 30 cents worth of coffee and danish because you are just not hungry for it later. Funny how we say such a protein breakfast "sticks to the ribs" meaning it has lasting power to conquer hunger. Lasting power it has, but actually it is the fattening carbo-cal breakfast that sticks to the ribs literally in terms of unwanted bulges. The bacon and egg breakfast satisfies our bodily needs longer, keeps the energy furnace stoked longer, and leaves our ribs unpadded.

It is better for a nearly starved person in a sub-standard economy to eat a bowl of rice to sustain themselves for another day, than to wait for a few more pennies for a morsel of meat. Nearly starved in that sense is a far cry from the nearly starved feeling that gnaws at you at midnight after a 3,000 calorie day. To the truly hungry, cheap carbo-cals are the key to life, and a potato a day can keep the coroner away.

However, if yours is not the famine stricken rice bowl environment, and instead you are in a more affluent "puffed rice" bowl environment, over-indulgence in cheap carbo-cals is equivalent to a death wish. And if economy in time or money is the underlying reason, you are really losing both.

Home, Sweet Home

By throwing the hot, white light of candid scrutiny on why you eat as you do, this book will help you to realize some of the factors that compel one to deviate from a balanced and nutritious fare. It is not always in the interests of time and money.

A 118-pound 22-year-old newlywed started to gain weight within a year of married life. A few months after the apartment was furnished and decorated, the scale began to move up. Her mother warned her of the perils of obesity and reminded her that her husband fell in love with and married a slim, attractive girl. It seemed only to make matters worse. The more her mother nagged her, the more she ate, and of course it was the carbo-cals that were handiest, and sweetest. Soon she was pushing 140 pounds and things were not as harmonious as they could be around the house. They had not celebrated their second anniversary yet, when she hit 150 pounds and at the rate she was growing, they wouldn't. In desperation she came to the author for help.

It was quickly apparent that there was more behind the craving for snacks and sweets than an active appetite. What happened after she started housekeeping? What part did her mother play in all of this? Discussions revealed that she had been very popular in the years before her marriage and had dates regularly with many boys despite obstructionary tactics from her mother. Flouting her mother became synonymous with fun. When she fell in love with and married her husband, her mother was all for it. The more her mother approved, the less fun there seemed to be in it. Furthermore, the quiet apartment days seemed dismally boring compared to the hectic activity of her single days. Her appetite for fun could be satisfied only by trips to the refrigerator or candy box. These trips became more and more frequent. Little did her mother know that by telling her to eat fewer sweets, she was making that indulgence sweeter than ever.

For some reasons that the medical profession have not yet fully determined, knowing emotional factors behind behavior of ill health is half the cure. Aided by this knowledge, our young wife agreed to condition her attitude toward her mother to a more understanding one. She substituted meats for sweets and joined a local bridge club to add some fun to her days. Her weight dropped 26 pounds in three months. Some time later, she also dropped the bridge club and became a busy mother.

Thousands of young married women soon have a love affair with their refrigerator. Reasons differ. A nation-wide organization called *TOPS*—"Take Off Pounds Sensibly"—is helping these women to regain their good figures. They simply meet once a week to analyze their *emotional reasons* for gaining weight, then help each other to restore sensible eating habits. Men, too, are joining *TOPS* for similar self-analysis.

Many people eat chocolates and other in-between meal sweets to make theirs more of a home, sweet home. Life can be full of bitter circumstances and there's nothing like a mouth-watering piece of fudge to make you forget your troubles, if even just for a few sweet minutes. "Candy is dandy," said poet Ogden Nash, "But liquor is quicker!" Both can be the opiate of unhappy people. The brain-washing effect of carbohydrate commercials and the sublimation of emotional locks are only two of many causes of imbalanced eating that leads to overweight. Among some overweight men, corpulence is a sign of opulence. The big corporation man pats his abdominal "corporation" symbolically. Sometimes a man that is slight of build, likes a large wife as ego compensation. A deprived childhood may induce greedy habits, or the same habits can be hereditary in nature. Organic disorders are lower on the frequency list in causing overweight than emotional factors, but they must be considered. So must causes due to physical inactivity.

This is a happy book. It will help you enjoy eating as you lose weight. And it will point the way toward even happier eating in the slender years ahead. It has been estimated that some thirty million men and thirty million women in the United States exceed recommended weight by at least ten per cent. Of these sixty million people, an estimated fifty million are aware of it and twenty five million extricate themselves from the obesity statistics and join the ranks of the hundred million normal weights? The answer appears to be that about half of those who diet manage to get back to normal at least for a brief spell, once a year, or brief spells twice a year. The other half never quite make it at all.

If you are interested in playing with figures about "figures," you can come up with some dramatic pronouncements like—there are about a quarter of a billion pounds lost and regained in the U. S. each year—or, overweight people in the United States have a surplus stockpile of over one billion pounds.

The yearning to be slender moves these millions to demand pills, tablets, and concentrates. Their demand has created new lines of so-called "low calorie" foods. New exercises sweep the country. Health salons and massage parlors help pound the pounds away. Yet the stockpile maintains itself at one billion pounds, a symbol of our affluent society.

As a people we weigh too much. And as a people we have not found out what we can do about it. Dr. Jonas E. Salk, discoverer of the polio vaccine that bears his name, is now devoting himself to research at his California laboratory directed at the whole person. In this age of specialization, the body seems to be divided into franchises with the nose, ear and throat man ignorant of the eye doctor's domain, and both in the dark about the adjacent specialized areas. There are skin specialists, bone specialists and—yes—fat specialists. It is time the whole person was viewed in medical perspective. Certainly the whole overweight person needs to be examined, not just his girth. Perhaps such an approach can yield for each person a pattern of overriding emotions and attitudes, physical functions and malfunctions that can be answered with valid adjustments and a permanent cure.

Meanwhile we can try to counteract the obvious nutritional errors of our society and know we are on the right track for everybody. One of these errors is an over-abundance of sweet and starchy foods in our present day diet.

How Much Weight Is Too Much Weight

If you are overweight, you can hold our high carbohydrate society to blame at least in part for the problem. If you are not overweight, you still have a problem—as you get older, it takes less carbo-cals to tip the scale and start you gaining weight. Eat as many carbo-cals ten or twenty years from now as you are eating now and your problem will be quick to appear. Meanwhile, our present high carbohydrate society is getting higher and higher, and the combined powers of carbohydrate suggestion are, at least subconsciously, hammering at the ramparts of your resistance. Mr. Apollo and Miss Venus are destined to become Mr. and Mrs. Fatten Easily unless they take steps *now* to substitute tasty proteins for tasty carbohydrates. It is a sort of future girth control. Chapter 10 goes into this problem of weight maintenance as opposed to weight loss.

Weight loss, however, is the urgent problem. Every year that you are overweight reduces your life expectancy. Even if you do become slender, and stay slender, you will not fully erase the damage that you do now by being overweight. In fact life insurance companies have analyzed their vast oceans of statistics on this and can tell you just how many years of how much obesity cost how many years of life.

At 35 years of age, a man who is 25% overweight for a number of years is reducing his life expectancy by as much as 12 years. A 35 year-old woman who is 25% overweight for a number of years is reducing her life expectancy by as much as seven years.

Suppose you are a man of 35 and 5 feet 10 inches tall, of medium frame and have weighed around 200 for the last few years. Your desirable weight is 160 pounds; you would be slated to live to the age of 71. At your present weight you are expected to live only to the age of 59.

Suppose you are a woman of 40 and 5 feet 4 inches tall of medium frame and have weighed around 150 a number of years, instead of the desirable weight of 120 for this age, height and frame. Instead of living to your full expectancy of 77 years, insurance companies will bet that you won't be around to pay a premium at age 70.

If you are more than 25% overweight, the price, of course, is higher. A man of 40 who has been 60% overweight can start writing his obituary now, according to statistical tables prepared from real life. A woman of 40 who has been 60% overweight a number of years has 15 years in her future instead of the probable 37 years.

If this is really a happy book that will open up ways to enjoyable dining without gaining weight, then why are we dwelling on these morbid statistics? The reason is this. Most people enjoy the status quo in preference to a change, even if it is a change for the better. Overweight people are no different from anyone else in this regard. It is easier to stay the way they are than to change.

The pages ahead will guide you by the hand to a better and longer life. But many will not go, preferring to take a chance that somehow the inexorable laws of chance will pass them by. A morbid reminder may be the nudge they need. Perhaps if they could see what lies in store for them in the years ahead, they would prefer to make the small changes described on the pages ahead.

Who can turn down a new lusty way of eating, when by eating the way they do they are courting heart disease, arthritis, and diabetes? Who can say *no* to a life of pleasurable gustatory partying and satisfying socializing spelled out in the chapters ahead, and prefer instead a chapter in their overweight life filled with risk of hernias, liver ailments, and inflammation of the gall bladder?

The penalties of overweight are a morbid, depressing reality. The fact that locked inside every overweight person is a skinny one trying to get out makes no difference. Those extra pounds court chronic illness as a way of life, make surgical operations a greater probability and at the same time a greater risk, and even exact their toll on mothers and their infants.

The change to a life of greater health, youth and energy can start by applying the first steps outlined in Chapter 2. The grim reminders are over. All the rest is fun.

2

Villain
Carbohydrates

The villain that puts pounds on you even though you may not be a heavy eater is about to be exposed. Mark him well. He has infiltrated your life. Now you must learn to take his measure. As soon as you learn to recognize carbohydrates and to count carbo-cals, the epicurean world of food is yours to enjoy without fear of paying with that pound of unwanted flesh.

Your reward begins on the pages ahead—gourmet recipes, international dishes, sauce secrets, appetizing snacks and tips for entertaining, shopping for food, and eating out—everything you need to begin your new life as a discriminating eater. Combined

. . . Unmasked

with your new figure and improved health, you will never want to go back to the old world of agonizing "diet" days.

Examine the two menus below. On the left is a typical day of sustenance in the life of a working person. You may recognize it as a doorway to the diet treadmill. Compare it to the one on the right. Even worse? You're wrong. If you were to gain weight with menu I, you could conceivably lose weight with Menu II:

MENU I	MENU II
Breakfast	*Breakfast*
Orange Juice (8 oz.)	Orange Juice (8 oz.)
Corn Flakes, milk, sugar	Two Fried Eggs
Coffee, milk, sugar	Four Slices Bacon
	Coffee, cream
Coffee Break	*Coffee Break*
Danish Pastry	Favorite Cheese
Coffee, milk, sugar	Coffee, cream
Lunch	*Lunch*
Club Sandwich	Martini
Apple Pie	Cream of Mushroom Soup
Coke	Chicken Salad
	Mayonnaise
	Melon
	Coffee, cream
Dinner	*Dinner*
Roast Lamb	Martinis (1 or 2)
Green Peas	Shrimp Cocktail
Mashed Potatoes	Porterhouse Steak
Gravy	Asparagus
Chocolate Ice Cream, wafers	Hollandaise Sauce
Coffee, black	Sauteed Mushrooms
	Tossed Salad
	Roquefort Dressing
	Strawberries, Whipped Cream
	Coffee, cream
Evening Snack	*Evening Snack*
Beer (8 oz.)	Cold Chicken
Pretzels (2 large)	Dry Champagne

It seems incredible, what about calories! The calorie count of Menu I is approximately 2850. The calorie count of Menu II is approximately 3250, or about 400 calories more. Yet it can mean weight loss instead of weight gain. Here is why: The carbo-cal count of Menu I is 1228. The carbo-cal count of Menu II is only 236.

This low carbohydrate menu is not just one-of-a-kind. There is almost unlimited choice in the world of low carbohydrate foods. But first let us examine high carbohydrate foods so that we can learn to recognize and avoid them.

Where Carbohydrates Hang Out

Carbohydrates generally wear one of two masks. They are either sweet or "filling." Sweet desserts, candies, cakes and ice cream are carbohydrate heavy. "Filling" bread, potatoes, rice and cereals are carbohydrate heavy. You will not have to give these up. But you will have to count the carbo-cals each time you eat them.

Let us take a carbohydrate look at Menu I again. Orange Juice is fairly high in carbohydrates. There are about 100 carbo-cals in an eight ounce glass. But, since this is a morning favorite and rich in vitamins, it retains a place on Menu II in our tomorrow. Cornflakes with milk and sugar add up to over 170 carbo-cals a bowl. Better not reach for the package to pour a second bowl. Compare this to the plate of two sizzling fried eggs and four slices of bacon. There is a grand total of *one* carbohydrate calorie on this whole plate! Feel like frying up another batch? Go ahead!

Menu I calls for coffee with milk and sugar. It has 50 carbo-cals, mostly due to that teaspoon of sugar. Drink four cups a day this way and you have satisfied your daily minimum requirement of carbo-cals and the rest may wind up you-know-where for all to see. Ever try coffee with heavy cream? It brings out the flavor of the bean to a rich and satisfying peak. Carbo-cals? A lowly three. Fill your cup again? Yes, please.

Can you imagine yourself being hungry for a second breakfast after this hearty Menu II repast? Hardly. But if you went along to be sociable, have some ham, or a few slices of your favorite cheese, or a side of sausage, and all the coffee and cream you want. You are not consuming enough carbo-cals to even bother counting. That fellow on Menu I having a fruit danish at the next table is adding 190 carbo-cals to his already foreboding total, and the day has only started.

A sandwich, pie and coke is the great American lunch. The sandwich with its two slices of bread (even whole wheat is 44 carbo-cals a slice) is more than 100; if a club make it 150. Apple pie is 200, coke 100, and the not so grand luncheon total: 415.

Let's presume Menu I belongs to a weight-conscious person who is making a valiant effort to "be sensible." The before-dinner cocktail is sacrificed. There's no bread on the table, no butter. He or she passes up seconds on roast leg of lamb ("I'll have a few more peas"), gravy goes with mashed potatoes but no seconds on either. Just one scoop of chocolate ice cream, and wafers. Coffee black, this time. ("That scale ought to dip, tomorrow"). Dinner was about 500 carbo-cals. Later, watching television over a ("just one") glass of beer and two ("take the rest away, honey") pretzels, the carbo-cal total drifts up to its final 1228 for the day.

Meanwhile, the person on Menu II has had a Martini before lunch and another one or two before dinner. There was intense enjoyment of the steak smothered in sauteed mushrooms and not one pang of conscience about the second heaping portion. After all there was not a single carbo-cal in the lot. There was no thought of holding back on the asparagus on which had been ladled as much Hollandaise sauce as seemed appropriate—two insignificant carbo-cals. Strawberries and whipped cream are 30 carbo-cals fewer than a slice of whole wheat bread. And why drink coffee black when you can drink it with cream, and without worrying about what it will do for your weight?

The contrast between Menu I and Menu II is dramatic indeed and serves as an introduction to which foods are high in carbo-hydrate and which are low. You are not expected to learn these values in every food. This is done for you in easy-to-use tables that start on page 110. Instruction on how to use these tables quickly and conveniently will be given to you later in this chapter.

How Carbohydrates Do Their Fattening Work

What is there about bread and pie and other carbohydrate-heavy foods that make them produce fat more readily than even fat itself? No simple universally accepted answer exists in all the reams of scientific treatises on physiology and nutrition. In fact, it is easier to find disagreement than agreement on just how the body derives its energy with various combinations of fat, protein, carbohydrate and material from its own storehouses.

One good reason that the issue has remained clouded up until now is that two people similar in size, expending the same energy each day, and eating the same food will react differently when they overeat. One will gain weight and the other will not. For some reason, the metabolism of some people will rise with over-eating, thus burning off the excessive food. But this fact provides no real help. The obvious inference is that drugs that will step up metabolism will also serve to keep a person slender. Such drugs exist and have been used for that purpose. Thyroid extract steps up metabolism and, by consuming more fuel, eats up body fat. But some bodies cannot long stand the strain of this increased activity. That strain eventually exacts its price on vital organs.

For people with steady metabolisms who fatten easily, atomic research has provided help in understanding biochemical reactions which go on in the body. Substances are "tagged" with radioactive isotopes so that their progress through the body can be followed. In this way, new information has been gathered on just what happens to proteins, fats and carbohydrates in the metabolism process. The results indicate that there is one villain, and one villain only, in the fattening process: carbohydrate.

This deals a rather final and crushing blow to the low-fat and low calorie schools of weight loss. It appears to substantiate the proponents of low carbohydrate schools, and there have been many. One of the earliest of these was William Banting, a fashionable London undertaker who included the Duke of Wellington among his clients. In August 1862 he was 66 years old, five feet five in socks, and weighed 202 pounds. Doctor after doctor failed to help him. He tried visits to spas, drastic diet, purgation, violent exercise to no avail. He could not tie his own shoe laces and had to walk down stairs backwards to keep his knees from jarring.

An ear, nose and throat specialist to whom Banting had gone to for ear trouble, Dr. William Harvey, saw immediately that Banting's ear trouble was due to obesity—not deafness, and put him on a special diet. By Christmas 1862, Banting was down to 184 pounds, and by August of 1863, a year later, his weight was a normal 156 pounds.

What was the diet that succeeded where all other had failed? Banting recorded it in his "Letter on Corpulence" published in 1864 in which he confidently stated: "Quantity of diet may be safely left to the natural appetite . . . it is the quality only which is essential to abate and cure corpulence." Does it begin to sound like he was referring to carbohydrates? He was. Here is the diet he described.

Breakfast:	Four or five ounces of beef, kidneys, lamb, fish or bacon. One ounce of dry toast. Tea without milk or sugar.
Lunch:	Five or six ounces of fish or meat and any vegetable except potato. Any kind of poultry or game. One ounce of dry toast. Two or three glasses of claret, Madeira, or Sherry wine.
Tea:	Two or three ounces of fruit, a rusk or two, tea without milk or sugar.
Supper:	Three or four ounces of meat or fish and a glass or two of wine.
Nightcap:	Gin, whiskey, or wine.

The diet added up to a whopping 2800 calories compared to the average modern low-calorie reducing diet of 1000 to 1200 calories a day. It consisted almost entirely of protein, fat and alcohol with an adequate minimum amount of carbohydrate and all the necessary vitamins and minerals that the body requires. It was low only in carbohydrate.

Banting gave Dr. Harvey full credit for his weight loss in the book which he published at his own expense. But the medical profession refused to accept that you can eat fat to take fat off, and Banting was denounced as a charlatan. His method, however, continued to be popular both among dieters and scientists determined to discover why it worked. The former were, through the years, more successful than the latter. Banting himself stayed on the low carbohydrate fare, kept his weight down and lived healthfully to the age of 81.

Many other experiments could be cited that took place in all parts of the world, all aimed at discovering a way to eat and stay slim. Many came just as close to the low-carbohydrate bull's-eye as did Banting. Others skirted it. From the confusion there emerged only one safe truism: Obesity was caused by overeating —by taking in more energy than was consumed.

It was not until 1944, in a New York City hospital, that a low-carbohydrate, high quantity diet was given a comprehensive test under scientific conditions, and the medical world took official cognizance and gave it the recognition it deserved. Some test diets exceeded 24 ounces of fat meat daily. Dr. Blake F. Donaldson was in charge. His work was so conclusive that low carbohydrate, unrestricted calorie diets began to gain considerable popularity.

In July 1956, confirmation came from the other side of the Atlantic with the publication by Dr. G. L. S. Parvan and Professor Alan Kekwick of the results of a controlled project at the Middlesex Hospital in London. Banting was right! Expenditure of calories in a person *increased* with fat and proteins, *decreased* with carbohydrates. A person could eat more proteins and fats, and weigh less.

Put Carbohydrates In Their Place

This is great. A person is no longer faced with starvation diets that frazzle the nerves and demoralize the spirit. All he has to do is switch foods around, soft-pedaling the carbohydrates.

But what foods contain carbohydrates and in what quantity? Can a person eat normally on low-carbohydrate foods or are they so rare that diet is severely restricted? Fortunately, it is relatively simple to recognize low carbohydrate foods. Fortunately, too, they are in very satisfying abundance in our economy.

The factor that will demand the greatest effort will be the changing of habits so that high carbohydrate foods are no longer king of the cabinet shelves. You will have to change marketing habits and alter your recipes. Menus will have to be watched carefully to prevent the culprit from infiltrating into every dish, every meal. This book will help you every step of the way. It will show you how to make the adjustment with the least effort, and the most fun.

In pointing the finger at carbohydrates, one must keep in mind that recognition is not tantamount to banishment. You can still enjoy your favorite pie or cake—occasionally. Many researchers, including Kekwick and Parvan, have recommended that 60 grams (about two ounces) of carbohydrate be retained in the daily food intake. Although even this amount will act to cut down loss of weight, it maintains a necessary balance and helps prevent any unfavorable side effects.

Sixty grams of carbohydrate, at four calories per gram, equals 240 calories. The round figure of 250 will be used to prevent a round figure in ourselves. The author has had person after person lose four and five pounds a week during the first few weeks on a limit of 250 carbohydrate calories, which we will call carbo-cals. There were no side effects. They looked better, ate more, and felt better.

With this limit, what carbohydrate foods can we eat? Well, suppose tapioca pudding was one of your very favorite desserts. Is it taboo? Checking our table of carbohydrate contents that starts on page 110, we find that an average portion of tapioca pudding contains 180 carbo-cals. This means that we can enjo one serving in a day but on that day we must limit ourselves other foods with just a trace of carbohydrate or none at all.

Taking the Villain's Measure

We must learn to recognize the carbohydrate villain so that we can take his measure in all the foods we eat. This means counting *carbo-cals*. It means cutting down, but not out, on some foods, going easy on others. All others get the green light—eat all you want.

What kind of foods can you eat without giving your carbo-cal tables a thought? What kind of foods require you to keep a running tab? And what kind are so high in carbohydrates that you must shuffle a whole day's menu in order to make room for them?

In Chapter 1 we discussed the main categories of low carbohydrate foods. It is open house on meat, fish, game, poultry, eggs, cheese and many alcoholic beverages such as scotch, bourbon, rum, gin, dry wines and some brandies. Non-alcoholic beverages include tea, coffee, postum, and boullion. Future chapters will give you many ways in which low carbohydrate foods can be prepared in unusual and exotic fashion. There will be ideas for desserts and snacks, too, which are hardest hit by the carbohydrate restriction.

There are sauces and dressings galore, including those made with cream, butter, eggs, cheese, spices and wines. You will be able to use your old favorites and many new low carbo-cal recipes later provided. This is not a once-a-day proposition as would be with tapioca pudding. The 250 carbo-cal guide permits you one or more of these "caution" foods each and every meal. But here is where you must do your calorie counting conscientiously— carbo-calorie counting.

It takes very few carbo-cals over the 250 mark to undo your day's selective dining and eventually be your undoing. By following its path through the body scientists have observed that radioactive glucose is converted to fat within three minutes after entering the bloodstream. Like any diet, the counting and restricting of carbo-cals must be done with accuracy and conviction. But unlike any other diet, you can eat all you want of delicious low carbo-cal foods and never have to suffer hunger pangs or conscience pangs.

As we read the table of carbohydrate contents, we enter the area where the greatest changes in our eating habits will occur. These are the high carbohydrate foods that have caused all the trouble in the first place. Know them by their starch and their sugar. See them in wheats and other grains. Mark them for what they are: human fat.

Pure, refined white sugar is 100% carbohydrate. Five tablespoonfuls would provide you with your whole day's quota of carbo-cals. Five times 45 equals 225. Remember this the next time you prepare a recipe that calls for a half cup of sugar (eight tablespoons, 360 carbo-cals). Powdered and granulated sugar are both 100% carbo-cals. Brown sugar is hardly any better, being 95%. Maple sugar is 90%. Honey used as a sweetener saves a few carbo-cals at 79.5% but if you use more of it you have lost your advantage. Maple syrup is 64%.

Thus everything sweet is suspect. However, if you are like others who have switched to low carbohydrate foods, you will soon look on sweetness as a namby-pamby pleasure compared to the rich satisfaction that comes with a properly blended Zabaglione, a mousse au chocolat, or strawberries and whipped cream.

Not quite as far down the list, but almost equally out of reach, are the flours that form the main ingredient for bread, cake, pies, cookies, crackers, and noodle and macaroni products. So anything in the family of baked goods is suspect. Let's see just how bad, and therefore how restricted they are.

While pastry flour is 78.5% carbohydrate, whole wheat flour is

72.4%. Buckwheat, potato flour, cornstarch and arrowroot are even higher (97.5% for the latter). One cup of pastry flour is 320 carbo-cals. One slice of whole wheat bread is 44 carbo-cals, white bread 48 carbo-cals. You can see how a slice of cake and a couple slices of bread can put you on fried eggs and steak the rest of the day.

An average serving of cornflakes is about 80 carbo-cals, but the sugar and milk bring it up to 170 carbo-cals a bowl. Cooked cereals, like farina and oatmeal are a little better. But watch out for cereals in general.

You will find that other food categories are not as easily tagged for carbohydrates as are the sweets and grains. Fruits run the whole range from a "go" on rhubarb, "caution" on melons and all fresh fruits, to danger on canned in syrup fruits and dried or candied fruits. Vegetables, too, vary from "go" on mushrooms, soy beans and cabbage, to "caution" on all fresh or canned vegetables except the carbohydrate—dangerous peas, beans and corn. Potatoes are equally carbohydrate high as are its root vegetable cousins—turnips, beets, yams.

Looking next at a few special foods: Nuts are in the middle realm. Eggs are "go" all the way. Fats and oils are fine. You don't have to bother to count corn oil, oleo, butter, peanut oil, lard or bacon fat.

If you have a general idea from these few pages of where carbohydrates are, that is all you need at this point. Gradually, as these pages lead you along the path to low carbohydrate, high enjoyment dining, and you measure various foods with the tables provided, you will become an authority on low carbohydrate foods and be able to guide others along this healthful path.

Some Do's and Don'ts Before You Begin

This book will lead you by the hand to a way of eating that will usher in a new healthy era in your life. However, the usual "shake well before using" precautions need to be stated at this time. Pay them heed. They may apply to you.

1. Any person who goes on a diet should consult a physician. Even the mode of eating spelled out on these pages is not a diet in the true sense, it would still be good practice to consult a physician, especially if you are seriously overweight and plan a sizeable weight loss.

2. Persons who are suffering from an illness should certainly consult their physician about any shift in their eating habits which they plan to make. This is common sense. There are some illnesses which would react unfavorably to a higher fat intake. The effect of fat on the cholesterol deposits in the arteries has puzzled scientists for 100 years. While the answer is being pursued by researchers, persons with hardening of the arteries should consult their doctor before changing their diet. People susceptible to ketosis should also consult their physician as they begin.

3. Start your new thinning process gradually. Sudden and drastic changes can shock the body organs. Shift your menus to low carbohydrate foods over a period of a week or more. Take your time. You are going to be slender for a long while.

4. Don't overdo it. Be sure you are eating at least 200 carbohydrate calories daily. Remember, this minimum amount is essential to your body.

5. If you are a compulsive eater who cannot resist food whether you are hungry or not and are extremely obese, chances are it is a psychological problem which needs attention rather than your diet.

6. A little bit of knowledge is a dangerous thing. If your friends envy your slenderizing results, don't give them a few piece-meal pointers. Lend them the book when you can spare it so that they can understand the whole procedure correctly.

If you have been one of those unfortunate persons who has been on and off a number of diets, a permanent blessing awaits you. If you have tried pills and purgatives and know how close to purgatory they can make you feel, you will want to shout this "discovery" to the world. The four main factors said to cause aging in women are overwork, excessive sun, fat, and crash diets. This book will not affect the first two factors (unless you take time off from work to read it in the shade), but it can end the third and fourth factors. Your days of crash diets are over. And your excessive fat is about to melt away.

The Right Approach To The Starting Line

A person who begins a trip, a project, or an event with doubt or confusion is standing in his own way. Success rides the wings of confidence and assurance. Past failures must be forgotten as you step forward the low-carbohydrate way. This is not easy for a person who has tried a number of diets only to be back where he started—on the scale. Take the lady in the following case.

CASE HISTORY A-4

For Her — A Last Resort

Betty, 39, was married and had two grown children. She was a nurse and the physician she worked for had made two or three obesity referrals to my office. Now she referred herself. She weighed 160 pounds, which for her was 35 pounds overweight. Being a nurse and close to a physician she had tried appetite depressants and diuretics over a period of four years. She lost weight but had developed pains in her ankles and wrists, which the doctor said was due to the diuretics, and she noticed heart palpitations, a symptom he said was often caused by appetite depressants. Now she would have nothing more to do with these drugs.

In examining her diet, I found it devoid of any over-indulgence. It was just a typical 20th century high-carbohydrate diet—one or two Danish pastries for breakfast, sandwich for lunch and the usual tendency to high carbohydrate fruits. We switched these foods with others: bacon and eggs, hamburger steaks, and melons—leaving the quantities and other foods just as they were.

The first week she lost three pounds. After that she lost two pounds steadily each week. When she reached 126 pounds, we added a half slice of toast with her eggs and returned some fruits. She leveled off. The whole process of return to normal weight had taken four months and not a single pain along the way.

This was truly Betty's last resort. Never again will she have to resort to stringent diets or to diet pills. The worst that can happen is that Betty may gradually let carbohydrates creep back in to unbalance her diet. The relentless bombardment to which our senses are subjected—the carbohydrate bombardment—will inevitably condition us to use these fatteners more than we should. The quieter voice of our better judgment is drowned in radio and television exhortations and the oh's and ah's of those around us who have succumbed.

But if this happens, Betty will get the warning signal from her scale. She now understands that all she has to do is replace some high-carbohydrate goodies with low-carbohydrate goodies. This understanding is a far happier condition to be faced than the despair that comes with embarking on another starvation diet that you know you won't stick to anyhow.

You, too, may have faced this despair time and time again. If so, not having yet had Betty's happy experience the low carbohydrate way, you may be inclined to look upon it with a sort of "I'll try it but . . ." attitude. This would be the wrong way, bringing about just what it visualizes—failure. Whereas a feeling of "I can" often brings about what it visualizes—success.

The author has dragged person after person from the depths of overweight despair to the peak of health and exuberance. I could do this only by leveling with the person—gaining a complete person-to-person understanding and mutual confidence. I am now going to level with you.

Let's have a heart-to-heart talk and see if there are any hidden doubts lurking in your mind about the low-carbohydrate way of

eating, about its being fun and good for you, or about your own
ability to lose weight with it. You pose the questions. I will give
you the answers to the best of my knowledge and experience. Together, let us see if we cannot sweep away all reservations so
that you can dedicate yourself with full confidence in success to
the fun type of diet that tomorrow will bring. If a question posed
below does not concern you, skip it and go on to others that
interest you more:

QUESTION: *I use sweets to give me quick energy. How will I get
this quick energy without sweets on a low carbohydrate
diet?*

ANSWER: On a low carbohydrate diet, your body will burn fat for
energy. You will get all the energy you need and as fast
as you need it. You probably need sweets now because
carbohydrates burn off fast, leaving you depleted and in
need of more sweets. Proteins and fats keep your furnaces
stoked longer. Furthermore, you can always re-stoke at
will.

QUESTION: *There have been a few books on the low carbohydrate
diet recently. Is this one any different?*

ANSWER: Several books have been published recently, giving the
history and theory of the low carbohydrate diet and listing some menus along with the U.S. Department of Agriculture tables of carbohydrate values. They are fine as far
as they go. On the other hand, this book is built on years
of experience with men and women who have lost weight
with this method and kept it off, with a minimum of effort. It is a how-to-do-it book, jam-packed with ideas and
techniques that will help you, too, to help yourself to a
happy, slender figure way of living.

QUESTION: *I have been told that low carbohydrate diets can cause
ketosis. Is this true?*

ANSWER: Ketosis is a form of acidosis. Mild cases can make you
feel queasy and liverish. It has resulted where persons
have been over-zealous and cut carbohydrates far below
the recommended 250 calories. Your physician will agree

that this minimum should be respected. If you are excessively overweight, say 20% or more, he may advise you to raise this minimum in the beginning, lower it later.

QUESTION: *Won't I gain back all the weight I lose when I leave this this diet, just as I have before?*

ANSWER: If you consider this a diet, the answer is yes. But it really is not a diet. It is a re-balanced way of enjoyable eating which you will want to adopt permanently. All it does is replace refined and manufactured products that are high in proteins and fats. Judging by others who have tried it, your dieting problems are over.

QUESTION: *I am really hooked on sweets. How can you be so sure I will have more fun on fats and proteins?*

ANSWER: You could have asked yourself that same question years ago about kiddie cars, tricycles, roller skates and bicycles. You outgrew these, too, and each stage led to a higher level of enjoyment, not lower. If you have been attracted to this book, chances are you are ready to drop candy, nice as it has been, and get "hooked" on a more sophisticated fare of eating.

QUESTION: *How do I know that changing my mode of eating won't be bad for me?*

ANSWER: If your mode of eating has kept you overweight, periodically or continuously, that is what is bad for you. Any sudden and drastic change can also be a shock to the body. This change is not going to be drastic if you follow directions, and one of the directions is *not* to make the change suddenly, but to make a gradual substitution of high protein and fat for high carbohydrate foods. What is also bad for the body is the repeated loss and re-gaining of weight that most overweight people experience as they go on and off diets. Changing to permanent low-carbohydrate dining will halt or prevent this damage to your body.

QUESTION: *Will I really be able to eat more and lose weight?*

ANSWER: You won't be able to make a pig of yourself *and* lose
             weight. But one thing is sure: You might be able to eat
             up to twice as many calories as you did on other diets and
             lose the same amount of weight. Furthermore, you will
             find proteins and fats very satisfying and satiating. Eat
             twice as much and it will feel like four times as much.
             And you will still lose weight.

QUESTION: *What about all this controversy on the so-called Air Force,*
             Mayo Clinic and Drinking Man's diets. Aren't they all
             low-carbohydrate diets?

ANSWER: Yes, they are. As to the controversy, it has mainly centered
             on their being tagged with Air Force and Mayo Clinic
             officiality, which both have denied. The medical profes-
             sion will argue both sides to most any diet controversy
             because not enough is known about the body's methods.
             A recent article in the Journal of the American Medical
             Association recommends a low-carbohydrate, medium-
             low-calorie diet with most overweight persons. The report
             is the result of a study by a team of nutrition researchers,
             Dr. Marshall Goldberg, Dr. Edgar S. Gordon and Miss
             Grace J. Chosy. The reason given is that what causes most
             overweight people to gain is a quirk in their constitutions
             that turns carbohydrates into fat rather than using it for
             energy.

QUESTION: *Is it true that high-fat diets can cause hardening of the*
             arteries and heart trouble?

ANSWER: This is a controversy that is still unsolved by the medical
             profession. Cholesterol, a type of body fat, was discovered
             to be present in cases of atherosclerosis, a thickening of
             the walls of the arteries said to be an underlying cause
             of most heart trouble. It was therefore thought that high-
             fat diets caused these maladies. Immediately, the word
             went out to get artery and heart patients off poly-unsatu-
             rated fats. But later observations showed that there were
             two types of cholesterol and the one that appeared to be
             the trouble-maker was not limited to foods, but was also
             produced by peoples' bodies. It was also discovered that

levels of both types of cholesterol did not seem to have any relationship with diet. All of this uncertainty is eclipsed by the unquestioned fact that you will lose weight on a high protein, low carbohydrate diet, and weighing less will be good for you.

QUESTION: *Is it possible that heredity has something to do with my problem?*

ANSWER: Yes, both heredity and environment can make us more susceptible to gaining weight. But neither can stop us from losing weight. The choice is ours, regardless of whom we are.

QUESTION: *Isn't this a fad just like all reducing diets?*

ANSWER: If it is a fad, it has survived longer than any other fad. The low-carbohydrate diet has been successful for more than a century. What scientists are not fully clear on is just why it is successful. Occasionally, the low-carbohydrate diet gets 'rediscovered" and enjoys a wave of popularity. The current wave of popularity might be interpreted as a natural reaction to the current carbohydrate craze that is making us fat.

QUESTION: *I am a vegetarian. Will I get proper nutrition on low-carbohydrate foods?*

ANSWER: Millet, soy beans, cheese and eggs do not lend themselves to the variety that meat, fish and poultry enthusiasts can enjoy, but you will find all your nutritional needs fully met in a balanced low-carbohydrate fare, for the simple reason that you will be cutting down only on low-nutritional, high-carbohydrate foods.

QUESTION: *I am sure I have some glandular malfunctioning that keeps me fat. What difference will restricting carbohydrates make?*

ANSWER: All the difference. As the pounds melt away, you will realize that the failure of starvation diets to reduce you was the diet's failure, not your glands! You will find that your tendency to fatten easily on less food than most nor-

mal weight people eat is more likely caused by your kind
of food (carbohydrates), not your kind of glands. In any
case, your doctor can help to chemically balance your
glandular system while making the carbohydrate "adjustment" perish.

This diet will succeed for you and it will become your
natural, enjoyable permanent way of life. There is no
question about this. Your physician, a century of experience in many countries, and thousands on thousands of
healthy, handsomely slender people will vouch for it.

Noted Washington journalist Joseph Alsop calls this the only
painless way to diet. After experiencing 600 calorie-a-day starvation diets and other weight-losing plans, Alsop, writing in a
national magazine, said that he lost two and three pounds a week
with a drink or so before dinner, wine with his evening meals,
and an occasional Washington banquet. Said Alsop, "I had found
a diet that is perfectly easy to follow at any time and in any
place, that can be comfortably resumed for a few days whenever
needed, and that always seems (knock on wood!) to work as
desired without misery or ill effects."

Noted nutrition authority Dr. Carlton Fredericks notes that an
excess of processed carbohydrates can cause many serious ailments. He endorses the low-carbohydrate way and calls starches
and sugars the real mischief makers.

But the most important endorsement will be *yours.* As you
turn the page to start Chapter 3 with confidence and expectancy,
you can count on more fun with food as you begin. And you
have nothing to lose but weight.

3

Enjoy Eating
As You . . .

George Washington kept a diary, now kept for posterity. It contains a number of entries on what he had for dinner or supper and provides us with a reliable record of the way some Americans were eating in those Revolutionary and post Revolutionary days. Here is what he had for dinner at a Long Island inn on an April day in 1790: oysters, baked striped bass, roast beef, stuffed veal, roast turkey, chicken pie, vegetables of the season, and preserves.

This was considered a "very plain and substantial repast" and Washington called it "tolerable good." Even presuming less than normal portions by today's standards, this plain repast probably

. . . Lose Weight

totaled over 2,500 calories. How about the carbohydrate calories? There were hardly any in the oysters, bass, beef or turkey. The stuffing for the veal probably contained about 50 as did the crust and gravy in his portion of the chicken pie. The only vegetables in season that Long Island could produce in April would be asparagus, dandelion greens or other leafy varieties as opposed to the high carbohydrate under-ground types. Add another 50 carbo-cals for the vegetables and about 100 for the preserves.

Washington probably consumed only 250 carbo-cals in this 2,500 calorie meal.

He was not exceeding the daily keep-slender limit, at least in that one meal. The percentage of carbohydrate calories to total calories is 10%, just about right for a good body maintenance plan. And judging by other gustatorial comments in the diary, he was not concerned about his weight, and he did not have a weight problem.

If Washington were to visit your house today, could you serve him such a meal? Sure you could, if you knew long enough ahead of time to make room in the refrigerator for all those high protein meats that you do not ordinarily serve in one day. You would have to plan specially, shop specially, and cook specially for what was considered in his day as "very plain."

As you now begin to shift your eating into high protein-gear you will find that you must change your shopping list, alter the nature of the foods in your refrigerator, freezer and cupboards, and revise your menus. You will undoubtedly have to abandon old recipes as you try new ones. But these are not the kind of changes that dieting has brought before, when you bought a package of melba toast instead of a loaf of bread, and when you reached for the skimmed milk or buttermilk containers instead of the richer products.

The changes you make now are more like asparagus for green peas, and chopped round steak for spaghetti, and cans of sauce,— you upgrade enjoyment rather than downgrade it. This is the blessing of the high protein, high fat diet as opposed to the high carbohydrate diet otherwise known as the "20th century carbohydrates unlimited." The high protein and high fat diet is good to eat as well as good for you.

How To Begin

In order to make a start in the home toward this shift in foods, a good place to begin is at the markets where you shop. Here is the case history of one woman who did this:

CASE HISTORY E-162

Che Cut Off Her Weight Gain At The Source

Dr. G, a woman psychiatrist in her mid-forties, weighed 235. She lived a busy life combining her practice with keeping house for her husband and three children. She realized that her overweight could prove a health risk, and yet found it difficult to hold to a diet and still set a good table for the family.

Her diet record showed an intake of about 2500 calories per day, 1600 to 1700 of which were carbo-cals. When I suggested that she hold to the same total but substitute 1400 calories of fat and protein for 1400 caloreis of carbohydrate, the idea occurred to her that she would make the change in the supermarket instead of in the kitchen. She bought eggs instead of cereal, cut down to half the potatoes, upped her meat quantity, selected cantaloupes and grapefruit for apple and bananas, and bought water packed canned fruit instead of regular syrup packed varieties.

It worked. The dinner plates had smaller portions of potatoes, larger servings of meat. Cake was served only to the children. She consumed the same total calories but only 250 of them were carbohydrate calories. She began to lose two pounds a week, then only one pound a week. She was cutting her weight down at the source—the supermarket. The last I know, her weight was under 200 and still going down.

You do not have to be a psychiatrist to swing your family away from carbohydrates by merely buying more of the other types of food. It is the simplest way to begin. It lets you begin gradually. In fact, the change may not even be noticed at first.

There are some tricks that help, and maybe a psychiatrist would be quicker to spot them than the average homemaker. For instance, if today you decide to cut down on potatoes, you should not have baked Idaho's. You should not even have baked Long Island or Maine's. You had better have hashed brown, home fries or mashed so that you can cut down on the portion without insulting Bill with the half-baked portion that half a baked potato would be. And if tomorrow morning you will cut down on the breakfast toast from two slices each to one or even a half, tomorrow morning is not the morning for soft-boiled eggs or fried eggs sunny side up for which a mop-up with toast is a ritual in most families. Make it scrambled that morning, well done; or fried over with the yokes broken. In this way, it will be easier to eat "clean" and the toast may not be missed.

Besides planning meals so that the switch will be less noticeable, you can employ the magicians' device of diverting the attention. Serve some dish that everybody loves. Or fancy up some platter so that it can't help but steal the show. Or serve large portions of meat and be over-solicitous on seconds. A show stopper or attention diverter, come hamburger-steak time, is broiled whole mushroom caps or heaps of sauteed onions. No one will miss the bread. At dessert time, if there is a chance that bavarian cream may be a let-down, garnish it with a mound of whipped cream. Then if you hear, "Mom, where are the cookies," you can reply with a cold stare—justifiably.

Your New Shopping List

It does not matter how often you shop, the next trip to the store is when you begin and this is how:

Following is a list of typical items on the average family's shopping list. They are arranged in probable order of their appearance at meals during the day, and on the shelves. If you shop often, you will be buying for fewer days, so your quantities will be less than someone who shops less often, say once a week for an entire week. Because of this, and varying size of families, no quantities are listed. Instead the terms *buy less, buy much less, buy more* and *buy much more* will be used.

Take such a list along with you when you shop. It will help you to cut down gradually in carbohydrates and substitute other nourishing foods in their place.

SHOPPING LIST

BUY MUCH MORE	BUY MORE	BUY LESS	BUY MUCH LESS
Melons	Grapefruit	Oranges, Bananas	Figs, Prunes
Cream of Mushroom, Asparagus, Celery Soups	Butter	Apples, Pears	Jam, Jelly
	Oleo	Fruit Juice, no sugar added	Fruits canned in syrup
	Cream		Fruit Juice, sugar added
Spinach	Milk	Cooked Cereal	Cold Cereal
Eggs	Tomato Juice	Pancake Mix	Sugar
Cheese	Consomme, Bouillion	Maple Syrup	Lentil Soup
Mayonnaise	Chicken Soup, Vegetable	Honey	Cream of Bean, Corn
Canned Tuna	Tomato Soup	Peanut Butter	Crackers
Canned Salmon	Canned Lobster	Apple Sauce	Pretzels
Bacon, Sausage	Canned Crabmeat	Pea Soup	Cookies
Ham	Soybeans	Potato Soup	Coffee Cake
Fresh Beef	Fresh Fish	Frozen Desserts	English Muffins
Veal	Cold Cuts	Frozen Dinners	Bread
Pork	Frozen Meats	Ice Cream	Flour
Lamb	Frozen Fish	Nuts	Cake Mixes
Chicken	Soybean Flour	Cocoa	Candy
Duck	Dessert Mixes	Cider	Lentils
Turkey	Ovaltine, Postum	Cola	Dried Beans
Mushrooms	Coffee, Tea	Beer	Corn
Cabbage	Ripe Olives	Potatoes	Peas, Yams
Lettuce	Onions	Beets	Cake
String Beans	Kale	Potato Chips	Pies
Turnips	Broccoli	Pretzels	Rolls
Cauliflower	Brussel Sprouts		
Onions	Carrots		

This list is not intended to be complete. However, it will certainly guide you on your first few trips to the supermarket, grocery, delicatessen, butcher or bakery. It will help with a gradual shift in your menus over a period of days in the direction you want to go.

If you are low on liquor, pick up a bottle of gin or vodka and dry Vermouth for your Martinis, or your favorite whiskey, but plan on drinking it straight, or "on the rocks." California red wine or a Chablis, Claret, or Chianti will be fine for dinner.

Remember, the purpose of a gradual transition is to avoid a sharp change. Do not expect to lose weight until the change is complete. The change will not be complete until you limit your carbo-cals to 250 per day. Even if you cut your carbo-cals in half (you are probably eating close to a thousand carbo-cals daily now), nothing is likely to happen to that scale. But then as you get in the groove on your menus and know how to recognize and figure carbohydrate content, keeping them below 300—watch the pounds melt away.

Take Stock Of Your Present Diet

A shopping list accounts for the regular meals you eat at home and perhaps some of the unscheduled excursions to the refrigerator and environs. What about the lunches in town, or the dinners out, or the coffee breaks at the luncheonette, or the occasional coke or beer? How do low-carbohydrate substitutes take the place of these phases of our eating habits?

In order to gradually close the door on excess carbohydrates, you must take stock of what you are eating now from the time you rise to the time you turn in again. There is a tendency on the part of most of us to gloss over our snacks as if they did not count. If you take an accurate inventory you may be in for some surprises. Remember, the purpose is not to eliminate these idle pleasures, but to *translate them to even greater enjoyment*. Once they are identified and their carbohydrate content evaluated, you can analyze just what ought to be replaced with what. As you progress along the chapters ahead, your particular eating habits will find exactly what they need for continuing them at a higher level of enjoyment. The blessing of the low carbohydrate way is that there are no habits to break, just new ways to carry them out and to satisfy them.

Here is what a typical 24-hour food intake analysis might look like:

TIME	FOOD	CARBO-CALS
7:30 AM	4 oz. glass of orange juice	50
	2 shredded wheat biscuits, with	145
	milk, 2 tsp. sugar	52
	coffee, milk, 1 tsp. sugar	25
9:30 AM	1 stick chewing gum	8
10:45 AM	Toasted English, butter, jam	160
	coffee, milk, 1 tsp. sugar	25
11:30 AM	2 peppermint lifesavers	20
1:00 PM	Cheeseburger	84
	Chocolate milk shake	228
1:30 PM	1 stick chewing gum	8
2:00 PM	2 chocolate creams	82
3:45 PM	8 oz. bottle of coke	100
6:00 PM	2 Manhattans	64
6:45 PM	Portion Roast Veal, natural Gravy	0
	Peas, mashed potatoes	100
	1 dinner roll, butter	75
	layer cake	216
	coffee, milk, 1 tsp. sugar	25
11:00 PM	8 oz. glass beer	40
	TOTAL	1507

If you were to analyze just the habits of the person whose record this represents, not the actual foods involved, you would see that this is a three-meal-a-day person who likes a quick breakfast and who eats lunch out probably at some type of a lunch counter. There is a mid-morning coffee break and a tendency to nibble in the afternoon and after dinner. Hard candy, chewing gum and an occasional soft drink are also part of the pattern. The total of over 1,500 carbo-cals will be cut to 250 by *substituting* foods, *not eliminating* foods. The habits will not be changed. The breakfast will still be on the run. There will still be a satisfying coffee break, the gum and hard candies, the drug store lunch, the afternoon nibble and the night cap. All will still be part of the daily habit. Nothing will be cut except the carbo-cals.

We have a problem, though. Is this a representative day, just like yesterday and resembling tomorrow? Or are we analyzing incomplete data, a day when things did not go just right, or a Saturday, or a day when we knew we were being watched?

The way to solve this problem is to record the same information over a few days. And, if we really want to do the job right, extend it to a full week. For many people, weekdays present no eating or drinking problem. It is the faster paced week-ends when a combination of food and drink add enough poundage to just about carry over to the next week-end.

Start your week of record taking now. It will not be a wasted week, for in the meantime, you will be carrying out a shift in your shopping list items and planning new menus based on the low carbohydrate items you are now emphasizing.

You can also be utilizing the alphabetical carbohydrate content tables that start on page 110 to evaluate your daily carbo-cal intake as you go along. Using these tables now for this purpose will give you practice in finding items quickly and easily and will begin to provide you with a better idea of what foods are the carbo-cal culprits, especially among foods of the type with which you yourself are having day-to-day experience.

Do A Carbohydrate Analysis Of Yourself

Your list of one week of eating should be complete right down to each lump of sugar, the last sugary soft drink and the dressing on your salad. With the carbo-cal values listed alongside every item you are now ready to analyze this eating pattern and pinpoint the trouble spots.

Keep in mind that the critical number is 250. This is the amount of total carbo-cals to which you will shift. It is probably more than the amount your body needs for proper energy and proper utilization of all the foods. It is probably less than your body needs to maintain its reservoir of fat, so you will lose weight.

If you are of average weight and stature, you are probably eating between 1000 and 2000 carbo-cals daily. If you were to also compute the total calories, you would probably find you are eating between 1800 and 2500 (women) or 2000 to 4000 (men) total calories in a day. At this time, you are not going to reduce this total amount, but you are going to substitute protein calories for the fattening carbohydrate calories.

Start by checking all items that count for more than 100 carbo-cals. These are the items that will require high protein substitutes. Using the one day example of a typical intake analysis given earlier in this chapter, the most formidable carbo-cal quantities arise from the shredded wheat (197), chocolate milk shake (228), and layer cake (216). They provide a total of over 640 carbo-cals. Bacon and eggs or another high protein breakfast is in the cards here. Iced coffee topped with whipped cream, fresh lemonade, limeade, or iced tea, are possible substitutes for the milk shake, but there are many other beverage ideas that will be suggested later.

The total carbo-cals of the three substitutes—bacon and eggs, iced coffee with whipped cream, and cream cheese cake: less than 70. But there are still over 1000 carbo-cals left and substitutions must be made to reduce them to 180, the balance now left in our carbo-cal account. This means that the next items in carbohydrate size must receive the same treatment: The toasted English muffin, cheeseburger, chocolate creams, soft drink, Manhattans, peas and mashed potatoes, dinner roll and beer. Do we eliminate them? Not on your eating and drinking life. Ever have a few slices of American cheese with your morning coffee? It goes as well with coffee as with apple pie. So do other cheeses; Europeans delight in the combination.

Would you trade the roll on your cheeseburger for one more of the delicious hamburger-cheese interiors, plus a side of lettuce and tomatoes? Any fast order counterman will serve a double cheeseburger without the roll, or double hamburgers (with cooked onions) without the roll, or two or three frankfurters (heavy on the sauerkraut) without the roll.

Somebody passed around an anniversary box of chocolate on the day shown. It not being a regular part of the eating habit, no substitute need be designated. But when you are carefully guarding your carbo-cal totals and the chocolates are passed around, you will not want to throw your total out of balance for the day and, instead of accepting, you will no doubt think of something complimentary to say as you pass them up.

Would you trade the sugar-filled soft drink with the low calorie variety? (Blindfolded you might not tell the difference.) Would you likewise accept a sugar substitute in your coffee? Would you switch from the Manhattans to Martinis or to whiskey on the rocks? Would you switch from peas to string beans and would you accept asparagus with hollandaise sauce instead of mashed potatoes? Would you be happy with a glass of hard cider or dry champagne as a nightcap instead of the beer?

If the answers are "Yes" to these switches, then the days of starvation diets are over for you. For you have just cut your carbo-cals down to 250 and there is every likelihood you will stop gaining weight and start losing it. What about the dinner roll? It fits into the carbo-cal budget, so enjoy it with plenty of butter.

Balance Your Carbohydrate Budget

There are scores of wonderful dishes and almost endless selections from which you can make your substitutions. The next chapter will show you how. It will give you ways to provide almost unlimited choices every eating step of the day from breakfast to nightcap. While you prepare menus and shopping lists for new dining adventures as you keep slender, there is only one simple thing to remember: *Carbo-cals must be budgeted.*

Your carbo-cal budget can be looked at the same as you do your financial budget. Seldom do men splurge on $20 white shirts when they are counting the dollars, or women on $50 perfume. That would leave nothing in the budget for other essentials. If you dearly love an expensive perfume, there is no reason why you cannot have it as long as you are willing to tie up the purse strings for a while. An ice cream parlor fling may cost you that dinner roll and a few other items on your expected menu in order to keep the 250 carbo-cal budget balanced for the day. Ever hear the expression "She has champagne taste and a beer budget"? Now it is reversed. Don't expect to drink high carbohydrate beer when you're on a low carbohydrate champagne diet.

Lest you think that a few carbo-cals over for the day does not matter, you had better prepare yourself for a surprise. Your bank will probably return a check marked "Insufficient Funds" when you overdraw your account a few dollars. Your scale will probably register over-sufficient intake the next morning if you exceed your carbo-cal budget by as little as 25. You may actually gain instead of lose, just by a small swing of a few carbo-cals.

There is no more dramatic way to prove to yourself the control that carbohydrates exercise over your weight than to cut them down to 250 for a few days, watch your weight drop, then put them back up 100 or 200 and watch the difference.

Figure A illustrates why the excess carbohydrates put fat on you so fast, while an increase in proteins or fats go unnoticed. The diagram is not meant to be a picture of what is actually inside of us, but it represents a symbolic picture of the fat storage process. Each container represents the amount of carbohydrate, fat or protein that a body might consume. As long as the container is not filled at a faster rate than the body consumes energy, the level will not rise. Eat more than is consumed for energy and the level in the containers moves up. When the level reaches the overflow pipe, the excess drains out into fat storage and we gain weight.

Now notice that the overflow pipe for the carbohydrate contain-er is fairly low, while the overflow pipe for fats and proteins are

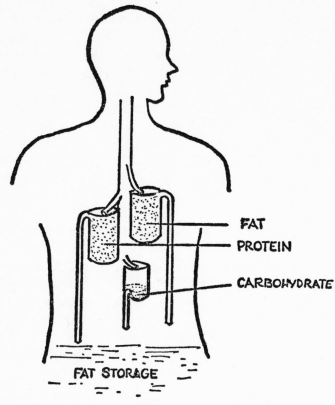

FAT

PROTEIN

CARBOHYDRATE

FAT STORAGE

FIGURE A

high. This means that when you eat just a little excess of carbohydrate foods, you will have an overflow into fat storage. Whereas, you can eat quite a bit of proteins and fats over minimum body needs and still not gain weight.

When you analyze your food intake and convert your foods to a low carbohydrate menu, you may want to count the pennies as well as the dollars. In the typical example analyzed in this chapter, the hard candy and chewing gum are in themselves only light offenders. Since it may be harder to change those habits than to say, switch from sugar to a synthetic sweetener, the chewing gum and hard candy are chosen to stay. You may prefer instead to substitute a potato or glass of beer for several of those minor carbohydrate indulgences. The choice is yours. *The only place you do not have a choice is in the 250 total carbo-cal count.* Let this go up and you let your weight go up and up.

Read The Labels

You cannot be a successful pennypincher if you have a hole in your pocket. Count your carbo-cals conscientiously and you will still fail to lose weight if they continue to slip through your security guard unobserved. Successful weight loss depends on an accurate carbo-cal count, and an accurate carbo-cal count depends on your knowing the ingredients of what you eat. A 4-ounce morning glass of orange juice might be counted as 50 carbo-cals. However, if it is the sweetened variety available both canned and frozen, it is actually 70 carbo-cals. This means 20 carbo-cals have sneaked in undetected.

Sugar may escape detection in a number of canned foods and frozen unless you watch the labels. Tomato juice may be sugarless but tomato cocktail may have sugar. Canned fruits and frozen fruits can be either water packed or sugar packed.

Federal law requires that the contents of all foods be stated on the label. This includes not only main ingredients such as the various vegetables in vegetable soup, but also the condiments and preservatives, if any. Since the actual quantity of each ingredient is not spelled out, there is no way to make an accurate count of a carbohydrate ingredient such as sugar. You would have to estimate by the taste what might be in an average portion.

Starches can also be exposed by label-reading, which discloses such things as cornstarch, flour and sorbitol. Cornstarch and flour are used as gravy thickeners. In that garb they can thicken people, too, if not counted in the daily limit. Sorbitol is a sugar substitute for diabetics. As such it is fine. But it is 100% carbohydrate. As such it is fattening.

In reading food labels remember the difference between diabetic and dietetic. Diabetic foods contain no sugar. That is the only ingredient that they strive to eliminate. What they substitute as a sweetener in sugar's place is the key. Most artificial sweeteners are free of carbohydrate. Others, like sorbitol, may not be. Your physician can identify a particular artificial sweetener for you. Dietetic foods can be free of either salt or sugar or both. Other dietetic foods are meant to be low in calories, so they will substitute non-carbohydrate artificial sweeteners for sugar. They are fine for low carbohydrate menus if you don't mind the slight after-taste.

There are many artificial sweeteners on the grocery shelves, liquid and tablet. If you hesitate on switching to one for your coffee because of an unpleasant taste experience in the past, try out several. You are likely to find one that agrees with your taste buds and has no detectable flavor of its own or after-taste.

Where some claim is made by a food product's manufacturer for nutritional benefits, you will find that labels are meticulous in detail. They list all of the minerals and vitamins, usually in terms of percent of minimum daily requirements (MDR), and often the total calories. Some will also analyze the food for percent or grams of carbohydrate, protein and fat. Of course, here our counting problem is solved for us, that is, after a brief arithmetical calculation of our own based on the methods set out as follows:

If total calories are given and percent of carbohydrate, multiply the two numbers and divide by one hundred to get the number of carbohydrate calories (carbo-cals). Example—total calories of a portion are 160. Carbohydrates are listed as 21%; $21 \times 160 = 3360$. Divided by $100 = 33.6$ carbo-cals.

If instead of percentage, the grams of carbohydrate are listed, you merely multiply by 4 to get carbohydrate calories. Example—total grams of carbohydrate in a portion are 41. $41 \times 4 = 164$ carbo-cals.

All of this arithmetic is done for you for over 2,500 foods in the lists that start on page 110. They afford a quick and easy alphabetical reference. The only arithmetic you need to do is add your totals for the day. If you don't enjoy adding, take heart in the fact those sums will not exceed 250!

An example of a thoroughly detailed label is this one that appears on an instant breakfast mix made with milk:

INGREDIENTS: Nonfat dry milk, sucrose, cocoa, sodium caseinate, lactose, extract of Irish moss, lecithin, vanillin and ethyl vanillin (artificial flavors), ferric pyrophosphate, vitamin A, sodium ascorbate, niacinamide, riboflavin, thiamine mononitrate, basic copper carbonate, and pyridoxine.

NUTRITIONAL ANALYSIS

	One Envelope (1.25 Oz.) Instant Breakfast	One Envelope Instant Breakfast with 8 Oz. Milk*
Vitamin B_2	24.0%	17.5 gm. †
Vitamin B_6	61.0%	34.0 gm.
Vitamin B_{12}	2.6%	9.4 gm.
Vitamin C	128	290
Vitamin D	26% MDR	35% MDR
Iron	25% MDR	27% MDR
Copper	20% MDR	30% MDR
Calcium	11% MDR	48% MDR
Phosphorous	**(.267 mg.)	**
Protein	**(.17 mcg.)	**
Carbohydrate	18% MDR	25% MDR
Fat	0% MDR	25% MDR
Calories	25% MDR	26% MDR
Vitamin A	**(.194 mg.)	**
Niacin	15% MDR	55% MDR
Vitamin B_1	18% MDR	49% MDR

†25% of the Recommended Daily Adult Dietary Allowance of Protein (70 grams) as established by the National Research Council.

*Values for 8 oz. milk from Bowes & Church, 9 Edition.

**No Minimum Daily Requirements established.

If a food's carbohydrate content is not determinable from either tables or labels, you may have to do some approximating from similar foods. For instance, the label of packaged "Danish Dessert" reads "Contains sugar, tapioca starch, currant extract, natural raspberry flavors enhanced with artificial flavor, citric acid, spice, U.S. Certified color."

Can you spot the carbohydrate culprits? Certainly not the color, spice or citric acid. Probably not the artificial flavor. But the natural raspberry flavor and the currant extract would have a few carbo-cals and of course the tapioca starch and sugar would be important enough carbohydrate sources to be counted. To approximate a carbo-cal value for this dessert use a value for a similar dessert that *is* listed. Tapioca is listed as pudding, with fairly similar ingredients, 180 carbo-cals, so this would suffice as a reasonably accurate value. Be sure to account for other ingredients, such as milk, that the instructions might call for. In this case, you add just water so 180 carbo-cals would stand.

Another dessert mix informs us on its package that it contains the following ingredients: "Sugar, non-fat dry milk, hydrogenated vegetable oils, precooked starch, gelatin, sodium caseinate, propylene glycol monostearate, adripic acid, sodium citrate, hydrogenated lecithin, sodium carbolymethybellulose, salt, natural flavor, U.S. Certified color, and BHA added as a preservative." Preservatives, flavorings, and chemicals can be ignored for carbohydrate quantity. Your dictionary can be helpful on some items of which you are doubtful. It will tell you, for instance that lecithin is a fat and you know fats are not carbohydrates. Gelatin is free of carbohydrate as are the vegetable oils. The items of sugar and non-fat dry milk are of course the chief sources in this dessert of the carbo-cal quantities we are watching for. Also, in this case the directions call for adding ½ cup of milk, 24 carbo-cals. Since the recipe serves four you would have only 6 carbo-cals per serving due to the milk. Add this to the carbo-cal value listed in the table for the usual gelatine dessert, and you get a good approximation.

On frozen dinners there is no need to study the long list of ingredients spelled out on the box. Just check all the foods as they are listed in the tables and add them up. Portions are average in both the tables and the dinners. Be sure to add values for flour gravies and breaded items. And keep a wary eye out for sugar which is often used in foods where you would least expect to find it.

Fulfill Your Need For Eating Pleasure

If balancing your carbohydrate budget means depriving yourself of much of your eating pleasure, chances are you will never really adopt the low carbohydrate diet as a permanent eating habit. It is equally important that you add as much if not more eating pleasure than you are dropping. We all look to dinner as a source of new experiences in taste enjoyment. If we are deprived of that enjoyment, it is only a matter of time before the best of resolves goes down the drain and we are back to our previous fattening regimen.

An important reason why the low carbohydrate diet is so successful is that it permits you just about unlimited eating fun. If you tried to gain weight while you kept carbohydrate calories to a 250 level, you would have to eat more than you probably would want. This is especially true when you consider how satisfying and long lasting a high protein meal is, compared to sugary and starchy ones.

The first principle you followed when you analyzed your weekly food intake and made substitutions was to try to keep your present habits even if it meant numerous coffee breaks or continuous gum chewing. The second principle is just as important: discover new high protein thrills in the world of food.

If this book is to succeed in launching you on a way of eating that will get you thin and keep you thin once and for all, it must show you the way to greater enjoyment than you have ever known before in the realm of the napkin and fork. This is what the next chapter proposes to do. In it you will be introduced into the fascinating world of the gourmet. You will learn many secrets of successful chefs, easy ways to turn plain courses into epicurean delights, hundreds of ways to diversify menus so that every day brings so many new memorable experiences that old memories of mashed potatoes and layer cake will be easily and willingly relinquished.

Later chapters will do the same for dining out at restaurants and will cover parties, snacks and fun eating for in-between meals. But, first, if you like to cook and are ready for some kitchen fun, put on your apron and come on in.

4

Cooking
For . . .

High carbohydrate foods are enjoyable to the taste chiefly for one reason—sweetness. High protein foods are enjoyable to the taste for a vast number of much better reasons: The limitless shades of new texture, flavor and new aroma that they can bring to you.

When the housing boom of the 1950's produced the living-dining room directly off a partially open kitchen, architects defended their economy-minded design on the grounds that cooking aromas are not to be shut off but rather should be permitted to circulate as a stimulant to the appetite. It is a good point. One wonders

. . . Pleasurable Eating

how much the charcoal and out of doors has to do with the enjoyment of a patio barbecue and how much it might be due instead to the prolonged aroma of the cooking chicken and the sight of the sizzling steaks. There is no doubt that food tastes better when the senses have been stimulated and your taste buds imbued with expectancy. In fact, there are some who will argue that the purpose of food is to bring delight not only to the sense of taste but to the senses of smell and sight as well.

One thing is sure. If the stage can be set for enjoyable dining, then there is less chance of the humdrum day and its workaday problems encroaching on a repast. Eating in harmonious, serene and attractive surroundings contributes greatly to enjoyment. The high protein meals you will prepare deserve an attractive and relaxed atmosphere so that enjoyment of them can be at its fullest.

Another important by-product of enjoyable dining atmosphere is good digestion. Frustration, discord and other distressing emotions are known to hinder the normal flow of digestive juices and the absorption of nutrients into the bloodstream. A blasting radio or television set, or a sulking child, may not dent the taste of french fried potatoes, but it can wreak havoc with the taste and bouquet of duckling "a l'orange."

Like the shift of emphasis in your marketing and the gradual change in your menus, the improvement of your dining atmosphere should be a step-by-step transition instead of an abrupt change. If the guest linens, fancy silver, crystal ware and glowing candles all of a sudden greet the family at some everyday evening meal, they are likely to wonder if somebody has gone berserk. It will not be natural and enjoyable for them, but rather seem like putting on airs or playing games. On the other hand, as each of your dinners becomes a new and enjoyable experience, the linen will seem natural in place of paper napkins, and other improvements will suggest themselves including, perhaps, some quiet dinner music.

Easy Protein Cookery

Lest the housewife feel that longer kitchen hours are in store for her the low-carbohydrate way, it must be emphasized now that the zest and flair that can be added to meals require no new skills and no additional time. It does require some new knowledge which you will find in this chapter and the pages that follow it.

Even this knowledge may not be new to many. It may merely

remind you of things about food and cooking which you have known right along but which have been pushed aside in the carbohydrate tidal wave that has engulfed menus in recent years. Is there anything new to you about omelettes and soufflés? Probably not, but you may have to be reminded of the many kinds of omelettes that can be prepared and a simple trick or two about soufflés. On the other hand, shirred eggs and eggs benedict may be, for you, entirely new ways to prepare an old favorite.

If you know how to boil, broil, stew, bake, (roast), poach, and fry, you already know the basic procedures that you will be using. If your family are barbecue fans, all your charcoal skill will serve in good stead for fresh air feasts. If you have steamed, browned, sautéed, and simmered, the simple steps in most styles of food preparation, that is the most you will be needing to do with even the most intricate and exotic dishes that will be suggested to you in this book.

The backbone of a high protein menu is meat. Other chief elements are fish, poultry, cheese and eggs. Before starting to give you new ways to prepare these and new types of foods, here is a checklist of these foods and what you can do with them. It will give you so much variety that you probably will not have to explore more adventurous dishes for weeks and maybe months:

BASIC LIST OF HIGH PROTEIN FOODS AND METHODS OF PREPARATION

Meats   *Methods*

BEEF

Beef, prime rib of	Roast, broil as individual steaks
Beef, sirloin of	Roast, pot or oven
Sirloin Steak	Broil
T-Bone Steak	Broil
Tenderloin Steak	Broil
Porterhouse Steak	Broil

Meats	Methods
Chopped Steak	Broil, fry
Filet Mignon	Broil
Chuck and Round Steak	Roast, pot or oven, stew
Corned Beef	Roast, pot or oven
Brisket of Beef	Roast, pot or oven
Other Steaks (club, chicken, cube, etc.)	Broil, fry
Short Ribs	Brown and pot
Flank Steak	Broil
Organ meats (sweetbreads, liver, tongue, kidney heart, brains)	Broil, fry, pot, stew

LAMB

Leg	Roast, pot or oven
Chop (rib, loin, shoulder)	Broil, fry
Chopped	Broil, fry
Breast	Roast, pot or oven
Rack	Roast, oven
Round	Stew

PORK

Spareribs	Boil, broil, pot
Loin	Roast
Shoulder	Bake
Chop	Bake, fry
Bacon	Broil, fry
Ham, fresh	Roast, boil
Ham, smoked	Bake, fry
Sausage	Bake, fry

VEAL

Cutlet	Fry
Chop	Broil
Round	Roast, oven or pot, stew

Meats   Methods

POULTRY

Meats	Methods
Chicken	Roast, pot, fry, boil, broil
Pheasant	Roast, broil
Squab	Roast, broil
Duckling	Braise, roast
Turkey	Roast
Goose	Roast
Guinea Hen	Roast, broil

MISCELLANEOUS

Frankfurter	Boil, broil, fry
Knockwurst	Boil
Bologna	Ready to eat
Liverwurst	Ready to eat
Salami	Ready to eat

FISH

Salmon, fresh	Bake, poach
Salmon, smoked	Ready to eat
Salmon, canned	Ready to eat
Codfish	Broil, bake, fry
Haddock	Broil, bake, fry
Trout	Broil, bake, fry
Halibut	Broil, bake
Mackerel	Broil, bake, fry
Swordfish	Broil, bake, fry
Bass	Broil, bake, fry
Perch	Broil, bake ,fry
Tuna, canned	Ready to eat
Herring, canned	Ready to eat
Whitefish	Bake, broil
Lobster	Boil, broil, steam
Crab	Boil, fry
Shrimp	Boil, fry
Mussels	Steam

Meats	Methods
Scallops	Broil, fry
Clams	Bake, fry, raw
Oysters	Bake, fry, raw
CHEESE - All Types	Ready to eat
EGGS - All Types	Fry, boil, bake, poach

In this entire mouth-watering array there is not one carbo-cal per portion with the possible exception of some of the cheeses. So, *there is no counting to do on any of these corner-stone foods.* They are probably already the building blocks of your present menu. Now they can be served freely and in many delicious new ways as you design your thinning menus.

Planning Low Carbohydrate Menus

Planning to put new zest into your meals is fun, especially when you stop and think that this is a reducing diet, not a figure-be-damned binge. However, it is also a responsibility. If you are lax about controlling carbo-cals, the pointer on your scale will give you the bad news fast. It does not take much in the way of excess carbo-cals to produce excess weight, as this young lady found out:

CASE HISTORY H-80

The Slices of Bread Turn The Tables

Lynne, 23, was a telephone operator. She lived with her folks and had come to me when she weighed 160 and was gaining. In several months she was down to 125 the low-carbohydrate way. I had found her to be a precise eater. She knew just what she was consuming, carried her carbo-cal tables with her, and tallied each day's intake. After she reached 125 pounds, she introduced her mother and continued to accompany her mother to my office each week.

Then she changed jobs. Her new job required her to bring

her lunch every day. Sandwiches, therefore, became part of her daily lunch menu. There were no changes in her other meals. In one month's time Lynne gained back three pounds. Those two daily slices of bread, 100 carbo-cals additional each day, were putting pounds on Lynne at the rate of 36 pounds a year. In a year's time she would have been knocking at my door again. Instead, when she mentioned the fact to me and pinpointed the sandwiches as the cause, I recommended that she freeze chicken salad or shrimp salad the night before, placing it in her lunch box the next morning so it would be thawed out in time for lunch. You can guess what happened. She stopped gaining; and even those three unwanted pounds had soon departed.

A Typical 250 Carbo-cals Daily Menu

In Chapter II, a low carbohydrate day was compared to the usual high carbohydrate day and you were introduced to an especially impressive day's fare. In Chapter III you saw how a fairly high carbohydrate day could be translated into the desired 250 carbo-cal day by a few rewarding substitutions. Now let us construct a typical 250 carbo-cal menu-for-a-day and use it as a basis for obtaining variations later:

Breakfast	Carbo-Cals
Tomato juice, half cup	20
Strawberries and cream, portion	28
Two fried eggs	0
Two slices of Canadian Bacon	3
One slice of buttered toast	48
Coffee, cream	4
Meal Total	103

You have probably stared at the two opening items which are to say the least not the ordinary way to start the day. But having a cold, tangy glass of tomato juice and fresh berries with cream is a lot more interesting than orange juice every day, and what is more, it saves five carbo-cals compared to a half cup of orange juice. You can substitute the orange juice if you wish but better go easy on the portion. You are better off having an extra slice of bacon than an extra swig of orange juice. What about a second cup of coffee with cream? Go ahead, there's room for it in the totals, as you will see.

Lunch	*Carbo-Cals*
Cream of Chicken Soup, cup	20
Chopped Steak and onions	12
Mixed salad, roquefort cheese	2
Low calorie soda	0
Meal Total	34

This is your lowest carbohydrate meal of this particular day. It does not mean it must be so every day. You may decide to have a sandwich for lunch one day and shift an equivalent of carbo-cals downward on two or three other items during the course of the day. Later you will be shown ways to construct a number of different lunches with equally low carbo-cal values.

Dinner	*Carbo-Cals*
Martini cocktail, one or two	0
Porterhouse steak	0
Mushroom caps, stuffed with cheese	2
Broccoli with butter sauce	12
Glass of dry wine	2
Cheese and wafers (3)	18
Coffee and cream	4
Meal Total	38

Late Snack	
Bunch of grapes	68
Evening Total	106
Day's Total	243

The home variations of this typical dinner are without limit. Note that the carbo-cals are low enough to permit an evening snack. Some people like to munch on a steak bone. Others enjoy a cup of tea or coffee with a cookie or two. For others a can of beer may be their "cup of tea." There are enough carbo-cals budgeted so that everybody from the fruit nibblers to cookie munchers can have their kind of nightcap.

If you use this typical menu as a basic structure, substituting to your own taste, you will eat better than you have eaten while on any diet, even better than many eat when they gain weight while off a diet, *and* you can lose weight.

Did you ever think that thinning days could be yours with nary a carrot stick or celery stalk in sight? If your friends poke fun at you about gravy being your favorite beverage, now the last laugh can be yours (providing it is natural gravy, without flour). Furthermore, instead of a longing, hungry "no thanks," you can take another slice of steak without so much as a caloric thought or upward flick of the pointer on the weight scales.

Start The Day Right

Food can become an obsession. You can enjoy a meal so much that no sooner do you get up from the table after one meal you start thinking about the next. This can lead to false hunger symptoms, as your glands react to your thoughts and carry out their pre-digestive functions. The menu-planner in the family is particularly susceptible to this. It is pretty hard to plan a dinner in the morning or early afternoon, visualize the ingredients, flavors and courses and not have your mouth water. The result: a trip to the refrigerator or coffee shop, even though you are really not hungry.

It has proven a valuable suggestion to many that this false hunger triggered by menu-planning can be foiled by doing this menu-planning before you have breakfast. If your shopping is on a day-to-day basis, do your planning for this, too, when you first arrive in the kitchen to put the coffee up. Make up your menu and your shopping list before you put the sausages or bacon on to fry.

Much has been written about breakfast being the most important meal of the day, and it is certainly a fact that it provides your body with the fuel it needs for a good part of the working day. Breakfast should provide you with both carbohydrate for quick get-up-and-go energy and protein for the long lasting satisfaction. That is why the basic breakfast you just studied has almost half of the day's carbo-cal quota. These carbo-cals are derived in this menu from fruit and toast. They could come from cereal, jams and jellies, or hotcakes as long as you budget your day properly.

Breakfast proteins do not have to depend on bacon and sausage. Fish is a very popular breakfast in England and other European countries. Cheese also frequents the breakfast table in foreign countries.

If you have tried to lose weight on a crash or starvation diet of 1,000 calories or less, you have probably gone without breakfast on one or more occasions, feeling that you are off to a good start for the diet day. A couple of hours later, weak and ill-tempered with fatigue and already a martyr to your cause, you reward yourself with a jelly doughnut and coffee. In so doing, your low blood sugar gets a lift, and so do you. But it is so temporary as to be downright fleeting, because here is what happens. When concentrated carbohydrates are taken, the flow of insulin quickens to help the body store the sugar as glycogen. So much of the sugar is changed to glycogen that very little is left in the blood. In what might well be less than 30 minutes, you are back where you started.

When a breakfast contains a predominance of protein calories and enough carbohydrate calories (about 100), the flow of insulin is normal and the blood sugar is replenished over relatively long time. If you are not in the habit of eating this type of breakfast and find it difficult to think about changing from juice and coffee, then at least consider using some protein concentrate, such as brewers yeast as an additive to the juice, milk or coffee in order to give yourself a well stoked energy furnace to carry over to lunch.

Eggs have survived the test of time as a superb breakfast food. They can become boring though if you pop them in water and set the three-minute timer every morning. Nor is there an adequately refreshing change by flipping them over in the frying pan on Tuesdays and Thursdays instead of serving them sunny side up.

It takes only 12 to 14 minutes to surprise yourself and breakfast companions with shirred (baked) eggs. Preheat your oven to 350°. Melt a teaspoon of butter in each individual heatproof dish. Break one or two eggs into each dish and bake 10 to 12 minutes until the white looks creamy. You can vary your shirred eggs by lining the baking dishes with chicken livers, cooked sausage, tongue or Canadian bacon.

Eggs Benedict is another interesting variation of an old breakfast favorite. Sauté several slices of ham in butter for two or three minutes. Place each on a piece of toast and top the combination with a poached egg and hollandaise sauce.

Omelets present another opportunity to vary the egg menu. Place a large non-stick frying pan over moderate heat. While it is heating, break three eggs into a bowl; add a tablespoon of water, some salt and a couple of drops of Tabasco sauce. Then beat to a foamy lightness. Melt a tablespoon of butter in the pan and pour in the eggs. As the eggs cook, stir gently in a circular motion; without scraping pan as would be done with scrambled eggs. When eggs are set on the bottom and still moist on the top, the omelet is ready to be filled and folded. Remove from heat and place the filling on one half; tilt and fold over top half.

Omelet fillings can be mushrooms, chicken livers, or jelly. A Spanish omelet uses a mixture of vegetables dominated by tomatoes, or a Spanish sauce. There are many more popular omelets. Be inventive—add to the list.

By combining eggs with breakfast meats, the variety is parlayed: bacon, ham, sausage, tongue, salami, liver, kidney. Eggs can be combined with cheeses, cheeses with the meats. Enter fish: pickled or kippered herring, salmon, shad or shad roe—and a long list of dinner favorites that also look very good to breakfasters.

Try eggs a new way tomorrow morning. Pick up some Canadian bacon, veal kidneys or country sausage to go with them. Then start thinking about expanding your breakfast horizons to new adventures in the days ahead.

Diversity At Lunch

Giving your meals a new dimension, will give you a new physical dimension, too—one you will be proud of and admired for. As you begin your low carbohydrate menus, you can begin to lose weight immediately. How much, how fast and how long will be up to you—and your physician. The next chapter will lead you along the downward sloping path of your weight loss progress chart and guide you in a situation that you may never have experienced before, a situation where pounds melt away faster than you have ever seen them go.

But the miracle of this will be missed and lost to you forever, if you do not capture the fun and excitement of high protein eating. For if you consider this a temporary way of eating, then you consider it a diet. If it is a diet to you, you will be off it some day. It is only a question of time when all the poundage you have lost will reclaim *you*. And if there is one thing that is harder on longevity than obesity, it is the marked fluctuations in weight to which people subject themselves by successive diets or reducing treatments.

Make a hobby out of planning and preparing delicious high protein meals. Follow the suggestions on these pages whenever you can. Be a sport about trying the untried. Then carry your new taste for epicurean dishes outside of the four walls of your kitchen to restaurants and parties.

The noonday meal provides an even greater challenge than

breakfast to satisfy the discriminating taste in a way that is at once quick and easy. The sandwich lunch is an almost certain casualty in the war against carbohydrates. Breaking the sandwich habit can be hardest for the working person who eats away from home. But it is also hard for the housewife who finds it clean and convenient to put a spread on bread, top it with refrigerated slices of almost anything, cap it with another slice of bread and bite in.

How the lunch counter can yield a quick, satisfying low-carbohydrate noon meal will be described in a future chapter. The home luncheon menu concerns us here.

Movie actress Joan Crawford loves to cook. It was her ability to cook that helped to carry her through her first lean years of road company work. Today the academy award cinema star cooks like a pro and she enjoys eating what she cooks. She is never faced with a weight problem and always looks her girl-like best. As you might guess, Miss Crawford never eats sweets. She starts her working day with a breakfast of fruit, eggs, pork sausages. Nibbles left-overs at ten. Has a noonday meal of steak and tomatoes. Enjoys chicken, chops or roasts for dinner. Sound familiar? Without actually counting carbo-cals Miss Crawford enjoys a low carbohydrate menu while still maintaining an excellent variety. One is not surprised to learn that when she feels hungry she enjoys a slice of kosher pickle—carbo-cal value, about two.

The first step of the ex-sandwich luncher is to have a sizeable portion of what goes into the sandwich, but with only one slice of bread. Cold chicken, chicken salad, tuna fish salad, tongue, cheese—almost anything that goes into a sandwich is appropriate on a plate without the bread and garnished with pickles, slaw, tomato wedges, lettuce. This is the second step. The third step is to provide enough dinner the night before so that there are leftovers that can be warmed over for lunch. Many casseroles and stews taste even better the second time around. Pre-school youngsters who have graduated baby food jars and have strayed with mother into the world of peanut butter and jelly sandwich lunches will welcome the change, possibly recognizing the occasion with "Are we having two dinners today, Mommy?"

A fourth step to attain the status of a truly sophisticated, high protein partaker, is to do as Miss Crawford does, cook lunch as you would cook dinner. How much more tempting to you and your luncheon guests than a hamburger between a mound of white carbohydrate roll would be instead little pyramids of hamburger atop hamburger, separated by slices of cheese and onion, and topped by a mushroom cap. No fuss, no exotic ingredients, no more work really than cooking an ordinary hamburger, but cries of delight from the kids and extravagant compliments from guests.

Loin lamb chops can be an expensive matter for dinner. But for your private lunch, they add up to plenty of enjoyment and no carbo-cals. The same is true of lobster tails or Alaskan king crab, both of which are to be found on most frozen food counters. And what about the whole family of less expensive but no less aristocratic soufflés?

The extra trouble and possibly expense in switching to low carbohydrate lunches bring ample rewards in maintaining an unbloated feeling for the rest of the day. You actually feel trim and vigorous. The world is with you and everybody is your friend. Funny what a difference two slices of bread off the noon menu can make in a day.

Five-Course Dinners

As you read this book and follow its instructions you will begin to lose weight. But, following its instructions can mean doing things you are not accustomed to doing, and ever since you were a child you have balked at change. Just about everybody has. Remember the time you had to be coaxed to taste something new? Then you liked it. If you can't remember that far back, maybe you can remember with disbelief having to coax a child to taste ice cream the first time. You have been coaxed to change your shopping habits so that you buy less sugar and starch and more proteins. You have been coaxed to drop most cereal and pastry breakfasts and sandwich lunches and try new ways of preparing eggs, fish, cheese and meat in their place.

Prepare to be coaxed again. Like the ice cream episode, you may balk. But then you will enjoy what you try even better than ice cream. And as you enjoy it, your weight will return to normal. You will feel better, look younger and function much more capably.

You are being coaxed to eat a five-course dinner instead of your usual three or four-course dinner. You are being coaxed to live it up with a glass or two of wine at dinner, if such can be your pleasure. You are being coaxed to try new dressings on your salad, new sauces on meat and fish, new herbs and spices, new international dishes, extraordinary thrills in ordinary dining.

What has all of this got to do with losing weight? Plenty. The incentive must be strong to successfully break old habits. Curbing carbohydrates must not be associated with a "diet," but instead with a different, more enjoyable way of life. In the past, the incentive of restored youth and health has not been enough to keep you on a measured starvation diet. Now, the incentive is not only restored youth and health but a permissive menu of delicious food. All you are asked to measure basically are bread, potatoes, and sweets.

Appetizer, entree, salad, dessert, beverage. First a martini to start things off. Later, a glass or two of wine to keep them going. Hearty appetite! The next morning your scale *will not* measure the conviviality and fun, the size of the portions, or even the fact that there were five courses. It *will* measure every forkful of mashed potatoes, every bite of roll, and the slightest deviation toward sweets and pastries. And it will multiply them many-fold, for these are the "*hooks*" that permit other foods to stick to you. The evening meal is the largest of the day. If you give it more than minimum carbohydrates you give it the "hooks" to hang weight on you. Without these carbohydrate "hooks," you need not have an ounce of concern as you enjoy yourself.

You are ready to seat the family. The adults have enjoyed their martinis; the appetizer is on the table. It sets the mood, from a champagne mood that caviar touches off, to the less elegant, but no less appetizing mood of herring in sour cream. The choice of appetizers with low or no carbohydrate content is vast. Chopped liver can be served a number of ways. There is shellfish—oysters, clams, mussels, lobsters, and crabs. Smoked salmon, pickled herring, and other cold fish make an apetizing beginning, as do mushrooms, egg plant, celery stuffed with cheese. A platter of thin slices of fine ham, rolled and pinned with tooth picks attract eager hands. Toast and toothpicks are carbohydrate. Get the message? Other ideas for appetizers and hors d'oeuvres are in the eating out and partying chapter of this book.

Forming the nucleus of your main course is the meat, poultry, and fish listed earlier in this chapter. But don't be satisfied with the simple broiling and boiling process. Try broiling on a skewer —like the recipe for skewered lamb on page 87. Try poaching instead of boiling—like the recipe for poached salmon on page 102. Instead of straight frying, brown and then simmer—as you do in the recipe for veal scallopine on page 78. And don't overlook America's contribution to cookery—the outdoor barbecue.

Sauce To Make The Meal Sizzle With Delight

Sauces add new life and piquancy to dinner dishes. You can marinate in sauce before cooking, you can cook in sauce, and you can add a sauce after cooking while at the table. Generations ago, the preparation of sauces for the evening meal started after breakfast. Today, with many of the basic ingredients available in stores, the housewife does not need to start from scratch and the time element is greatly reduced. Most sauces start with these ingredients: wine, cream, ketchup, mayonnaise, tomato puree, wine vinegar, Worcester sauce, anchovy essence, and salad oil. To one or more of these you will be adding dried herbs, pepper, salt and other seasonings. A number of recipes for sauces and entrees using sauces are up ahead a few pages. Sauces afford unhurried moments of fun time in the kitchen and can make all the difference between eating and dining. Sauces are particularly helpful in making the vegetable portions of your entree hold its own with the feature performer. You will be working mostly with mushrooms, cabbage, asparagus, soy beans, spinach, celery, tomatoes, chard, broccoli and greens of all types. Sauces become dressings applied to salad. No carbo-cal counting to speak of for French, Russian, Roquefort, Mayonnaise or any of the vinegar and oil dressings.

Foreign Lessons In Low Carbohydrate Cookery

Nothing is as impressive to family or guests, and gustatorially satisfying to yourself, as a zesty dish from a foreign land. Europeans and orientals are not better cooks, but they do things in the kitchen differently, often with the same ingredients. It is the difference that scores. A dish does not have to be impractical to be exotic. In fact, you will admire the ingenuity of cooks in other lands as you savour new subtle flavors derived from familiar ingredients, newly wed.

Here you will have to avoid many of the starchy elements, for they, too, are universal. Visitors to Austria often gain weight, mostly due to the bread crumbs and flour in most recipes, not to speak of the irresistible Austrian pastries. (Their chicken paprika is delicious and just about carbohydrate free.) Even Chinese food can be carbohydrate-heavy due to the cornstarch thickening in many of their dishes. On the other hand, Japanese seldom, if ever, use cornstarch. See their chicken teriyaki recipe on page 83, or the standard suki-yaki.

The list of internationally famous recipes made up of ingredients with zero to a trace of carbohydrate is too extensive for you to cover in a lifetime, even though you live many years longer by their grace. A scattering are given in the menu section ahead, but a long list of recipe books are available to the adventuresome. Count your carbohydrates by estimating the value of carbohydrate foods that must enter the recipe. If a quarter of a cup of flour is called for in a recipe for six, this means you are charged with 84 divided by six or 16 carbo-cals.

In many interesting new entrees from Thailand, France, Holland, India, Syria and other far away countries you will find the carbohydrate count is zero. You will also find new ways to prepare vegetables, too, and even low-carbohydrate desserts. Salads become spice hot in Korea and yogurt bland in the Middle East. Fish is eaten in Japan and Polynesia only after it is first marinated in fruit juices or vinegars which in effect cook them and make them entirely acceptable to the American table. A favorite dessert in France is cheese and crackers. The French are also the source for wine and herb cooking techniques that have made them famous and French cookbooks reveal their skills of the skillet. Favorite vegetables in Italy are dandelion greens, fennuchio (anise-flavored) and scallions, but carbo-cal counters can go bankrupt on their spaghettis, macaronis, and other dry dough pastas. Many home gardens are growing exotic Chinese vegetables such as snow peas and Chinese cabbage, seen more frequently now, too, in vegetable store bins and frozen food counters. Denmark is famous for hors d'oeuvres chiefly of shellfish and cheeses, and these alone merit our forgiveness for their namesake pastry to which we owe so much of our waistline.

Low Carbohydrate Desserts

The greatest challenge that awaits you is devising low-carbohydrate desserts. Flour-less and sugar-less, it would seem a dessert by any name could never taste as sweet. The average cake, ice cream, pastry and pudding dessert runs from 150 to 300 carbo-cals. To include an average portion of apple pie, 210 carbo-cals, in your day's budget would freeze out other foods like orange juice and fresh vegetables which contain important nutrients. There is not exactly a nevermore about it, because one day's nutrients will not be missed, but there is most certainly a hardly-ever-more.

What can the carbo-cal budget stand for dessert? Shoot for 60 to 100 carbo-cals, depending on the rest of the day's menu. Of course this excludes pastry. Even a cupcake or slice of plain sponge cake will saturate your dinner with enough carbo-cals as to wreak havoc with the scale. If you can be satisfied with one oatmeal cookie or brownie, fine—but can you!

All is not lost. There are many dessert ingredients on our list of "go" foods—and others that are fairly low in carbohydrates: butter, cream, and eggs; many fruits and most berries; essences and flavorings such as cinnamon and vanilla; and some nuts.

As a result we find the following desserts available in our menu planning:

DESSERT	PORTION QUANTITY	ESTIMATED CARBO-CALS PER PORTION
Jello (or similar)	½ cup	64
Jello-O Whipped Dessert	½ cup	80
Fruit Cake	½ slice	75
Sugar Wafers	2 large	72
Raw Apple	medium	64
Raw Cherries	1 cup	60
Grapefruit	medium half	72
Banana custard with meringue	1 cup	76
Banana Whip	½ cup	62

DESSERT	PORTION QUANTITY	ESTIMATED CARBO-CALS PER PORTION
Butterscotch (sugar-free mix) pudding	½ cup	36
Junket	½ cup	20
Rice pudding	½ cup	68
Banana and cream	one medium	85
Blueberries and cream	⅔ cup	65
Raspberries and cream	⅔ cup	68
Strawberries and cream	⅔ cup	36
Cantaloupe	one half, medium	32
Guava	one medium	60
Honeydew melon	average slice	32
Peaches, sliced fresh and cream	one large	74
Pineapple, fresh	⅔ cup, diced	50
Watermelon	1″ by 8″ by 10″	52
Custard	¾ cup	90
Chiffon pudding	¾ cup	70
Bavarian Cream	¾ cup	80
Chocolate mousse	½ cup	60
Biscuit tortoni	1 oz. cup	70
Floating Island	¾ cup	60

The list is by no means complete, but it is appetizing. If you use artificial sweeteners, you can add to the list and also the size of portions. Some non-sweet liqueurs, like Kirsch, can be added to fruit for diversity. A thin Swedish pancake (crepes suzette) with a teaspoon of jelly just about makes an 80 or 90 carbo-cal budget. Check the avacado dessert on page 107. It is simply delicious. There are many more variations of the above which can be created with a little low-carbohydrate ingenuity.

Top off your dinner with tea or coffee. Experiment with new teas and new blends of coffee which you grind from the bean (mechanical blenders are good coffee grinders). The sugar must go. It is 16 carbo-cals per teaspoon. If fresh sweet cream does not sweeten it enough for you, use an artificial sweetener. Try out several until you find one that suits your taste.

In the section that follows this chapter are the reference tables, charts and menus that will guide you in the world of low-carbohydrate foods. Use them to help you in the first two steps of your gradual shift to high protein foods—marketing and menu planning. The next chapter will assume that you have made a start on your gradual shift. It will tell you what to expect from your scale now, and how to ride its pointer down to your proper weight.

HIGH-PROTEIN RECIPES

Entrees

CHICKEN ITALIAN STYLE

3 lb. Broiler
1 cup minced onion
1 large green or red pepper
    chopped
½ cup wine
1 small can tomato paste
1 garlic clove

1 large can tomatoes or about
    5 medium-fresh tomatoes
½ cup salad or olive oil
2 bay leaves
salt
½ tsp. oregano
½ tsp. basil

In dutch oven heat oil and brown chicken. Add 1 clove garlic, remove when browned and discard. Add chopped vegetables and lightly brown, add all other ingredients and cook over low heat for about 45 minutes. Serves 6

BARBECUED CHICKEN

Marinate cut-up chicken or chicken parts in:
½ cup soy sauce
½ cup ketchup
Juice of 1 lemon
Touch of sugar

Let remain for a couple of hours. Baste chicken as it broils. To speed outdoor cooking time, broil five minutes each side in oven first.

STEAK ALFREDO

Marinate sirloin steak in red cooking wine and 3 garlic cloves. In a little oil, brown 1 sliced red, hot pepper (seeds removed), 1 sliced medium onion, ½ lb. sliced mushrooms. Add a touch of red wine and a dash of good soy sauce. Cut up steak into cubes, heat in sauce and serve.

VEAL SCALLOPINE

2 lbs. thinly sliced and pounded veal
4 sliced fresh tomatoes
3 tbs. olive oil
½ lb. fresh mushrooms
2 garlic cloves
½ cup white wine
fresh parsley
seasoning

In large frying pan brown veal quickly with garlic. Remove garlic, discard. Remove veal. Brown mushrooms several minutes. Replace veal, add remaining ingredients and simmer covered until tender, between 5 and 10 minutes. Serves 8.

MEAT LOAF SUPREME

1 lb. lean chopped beef
½ lb. chopped pork or veal
½ cup each finely chopped onion, celery and carrot simmered first
in 1 cup beef stock until almost tender.

Marinate ground meat in ⅔ cup red wine. Season with dash Worcester, salt and pepper to taste. Shape in leaf pan and cook at 350° for 30-40 minutes. Serves 5-6.

BROILED FLANK STEAK

3 lbs. flank steak
1½ garlic clove, sliced
1 tbs. soy sauce
2 tbs. red wine
1 tsp. sugar

Mix above ingredients and marinate steak at room temperature for 2 hours or more. Broil 7 minutes on first side and 5 minutes on reverse side. Slice thinly against the grain. Serves 8

LOBSTER SCAMPI

6 Rock Lobster tails defrosted with soft undershell removed
¾ cup oil
iuice of small lemon

¾ tsp. salt
⅛ tsp. pepper
several sprigs fresh chopped parsley
2 large minced garlic cloves

Marinate tails in remaining ingredients for about 1 hour, turning a few times. Broil shell side up dotted with butter. Serve with marinade.

PATIO TUNA AND SHRIMP

Toss 2 cans white meat tuna with mayonnaise. Add ½ lb. cooked and cooled shrimps. Add more mayonnaise, pepper and a touch of dried tarragon. Serve cold on lettuce.

SALMON RING A LA REINE

Remove skin and bones from 2 cans salmon. Place in bowl and add 1½ cups finely diced celery, 1 cup mayonnaise, ½ cup sweet pickle (optional), 2 tbs. chopped onions, 2 tbs. lemon juice, 1 tbs. Worcester sauce, ¾ - 1 tbs. salt. Mix together. Dissolve 1 envelope plain gelatin in ¼ cup cold water, let stand 5 minutes then heat with ½ cup boiling water until thoroughly blended. Fold gelatin into salmon. Lightly rub ring mold with salad oil. Fill with mixture and chill until firm. Remove from mold and garnish with parsley.
Serve with Avocado dressing:
Peel and remove seed from medium Avocado. Mash and stir in 1 cup sour cream, ½ cup mayonnaise, 1 tbs. lemon juice and ½ tsp. horseradish.

FILLETS OF FISH IN WINE

1 lb. fish fillets, frozen or fresh
1 tbs. margarine
1 onion, chopped
1 garlic clove minced
1 tbs. chopped parsley
1 medium can tomatoes
½ cup white wine
dash oregano or tarragon
2 tbs. cream
salt and pepper to taste.

Cut fillets in half. Melt margarine in frying pan and brown onion and garlic until golden. Place fish in pan, covered by tomatoes, wine and parsley. Heat to boiling, cover and simmer about 15 minutes. Add oregano and blend in cream, stirring until smooth. Serve garnished with parsley. Serves 4

BRAISED SHORT RIBS OF BEEF

3 lbs. short ribs of beef (cut 3" long)
4 tbs. flour
3 tbs. salt
½ tsp. black pepper
2 tbs. shortening or oil
2 cups bouillon
6 medium sized onions (white)
5 celery stalks
½ tsp. thyme leaves
½ bay leaf
2 tbs. cold water

Trim excess fat from beef. Combine 3 tbs. of flour with salt and pepper and dip meat into this mixture. Brown meat on all sides in shortening or oil in deep pan. Add bouillon, cover and simmer for two hours or until meat is tender. Add onion and cook for ten more minutes, covered. Cut celery into strips 2 inches long and add to above. Add the thyme, bay leaf and cover, cook for 25 minutes more, until vegetables are soft. Remove meat and vegetables. Combine the remaining flour and water and stir into the simmering gravy. After the gravy has thickened, cook for one minute and serve with meat and vegetables. Serves six to eight.

WINEGROWER'S BEEF

3 lbs. cubed chuck or top round
2 cups red Bordeaux wine
1 tsp. thyme
1 crushed bay leaf
1 tbs. oil
1 sliced carrot
2 sprigs parsley
1 onion sliced

2 tbs. shortening
2 tbs. flour
1 cup consomme
2 cloves crushed garlic
pinch salt
¼ lb. diced salt pork
1 doz. small white onions
2 tbs. chopped onions

Marinate beef overnight in mixture of wine, thyme, bay leaf, oil, carrot, parsley and sliced onion. Drain. Save marinade after it has been strained. Place shortening in dutch oven and heat. Brown meat on all sides, add chopped onions and cook until slightly brown. Add flour and stir until brown. Add consomme, marinade, garlic and salt, stirring until it comes to a boil. Cover and let simmer for half an hour. Cook pork until brown. Remove from pan. Cook onions in pork fat until brown. To beef mixture, add pork and onions, and simmer, covered for about two hours or until meat is tender. Serves six

CHICKEN IN WINE

2 small broilers
cup melted butter
1 tsp. salt
pinch pepper
paprika
monosodium glutamate
1 cup Sherry or Madeira wine

Have broilers cut in half. Brush with melted butter, and sprinkle with salt, pepper, paprika, monosodium glutamate and broil on both sides until slightly brown. Pour more melted butter and wine over them. Now place pan in oven and cover. Baste the chicken 2 or 3 times during the half hour baking time in a medium hot oven.

INDONESIAN PORK

2 lbs. lean pork
1 cup salted peanuts
2 tbs. finely ground coriander
seeds
2 cloves minced garlic
crushed red pepper
3 medium sized onions
chopped

3 tbs. lemon juice
2 tbs. brown sugar
¼ cup soy sauce
black pepper
½ cup melted butter
½ cup water or chicken
flavored bouillon

Trim all fat from pork. Cut into cubes. With all the ingredients except for the melted butter and chicken bouillon, make a puree in an electric blender. Pour this into saucepan and bring to a boil. Now add the melted butter and bouillon. Let mixture cool and pour over the pork. Let this stand one or two hours. Place the meat

on skewers and cook over charcoal. Baste occasionally with sauce.
If you have any sauce leftover, reheat it and serve with the meat.
Serves six

TANGY TUNA RING

1 can flaked tuna (drained)	2 tbs. catsup
2 tbs. lemon juice	1 tbs. salt
1 tbs. unflavored gelatin	½ chopped green pepper
½ cup cold water	4 or 5 chopped celery stalks
½ pint sour cream	

Sprinkle lemon juice over tuna. Dissolve gelatin over hot water
after softening it in cold water. Let it cool slightly. Stir in tuna,
sour cream, catsup, salt, green pepper and celery. Pour into a
3-cup ring mold. Chill until firm and unmold. Can be served with
lemon wedges. Serves 4

CORNED-BEEF LOAF

1 tbs. unflavored gelatin	1 can corned beef (crumbled)
¼ cup cold water	12 ozs.
12 ozs. heated tomato juice	½ cup chopped celery
2 tsp. lemon juice	1 medium cucumber chopped
½ tsp. salt	chopped onion to taste
	1 cup mayonnaise

Soften gelatin in cold water, then dissolve in hot tomato juice.
Add lemon juice and salt and chill until slightly set. Stir in corned
beef, celery, cucumber, onion and mayonnaise and chill until firm
in a loaf pan (1½x4½x2½). Unmold on crisp lettuce and trim with
cucumber slices and serve with hardboiled eggs or deviled eggs.
Serves 8

HAM AND CHEESE MOLD

1 pkg. gelatin (lemon flavored)	2 drops Tabasco sauce
1 cup hot water	1 cup cooked or canned ham (diced)
½ cup cold water	½ cup sharp American cheese (shredded)
½ cup mayonnaise	¼ cup green pepper (diced)
2 tsp. vinegar	2 tbs. pimiento (diced)
1½ tsp. horseradish	grated onion to taste
pinch salt	

Dissolve gelatin in hot water and add cold water, mayonnaise, vinegar, horseradish, salt and Tabasco sauce. Blend well and pour into refrigerator tray. Chill in freezing unit for 20 minutes or until firm about 1 inch from edge, but still soft in center. Turn into bowl and beat until light and fluffy. Fold in remaining ingredients and pour into a one quart mold. Chill for 30 to 60 minutes or until firm. Unmold and serve. Serves 6

CHICKEN TERIYAKI

Cut up chicken fryer in small pieces and marinate and broil with the bones to eat with fingers like spareribs. Or remove bones from parts of a 2½ lb. fryer or use 3 chicken breasts and de-bone. Cut chicken in small pieces and thread on skewers. Marinate for 2 hours in:

⅔ cup soy oil
⅓ cup dry white wine, sherry or vermouth
1 clove minced garlic
⅛ tbs. ground ginger
1 tbs. sugar

CHICKEN CURRY

3 small onions
3 tbs. soy oil
1 tbs. curry powder
1 medium chicken, cut into small pieces
1 cup hot water or vegetable cooking juice

Slice onions and fry to golden brown in the hot oil. Remove and set aside. Add curry powder to oil (add more if necessary) and stir. Add chicken pieces and brown. Chop cooked onion, add to chicken and cover with hot water or vegetable juice, simmer covered for about one hour.

LAMB RAGOUT

2 lbs. lean lamb cut in 1"
   cubes
½ tsp. salt
freshly ground pepper
¼ cup olive oil

1 can consomme undiluted
⅓ cup sherry
1 clove garlic, minced
2 tbs. lemon juice
2 tbs. chopped fresh parsley

Season meat. Heat oil and brown lamb on all sides, in the heated oil. Add consomme, sherry and garlic, and heat. Cover the pan and cook until tender, about one hour. Stir in the lemon juice and sprinkle with parsley.

BEEF & TOMATOES

1 lb. lean beef (round, sirloin or flank steak)
4 to 6 medium-size tomatoes
4 to 6 medium-size onions
1 small slice of raw ginger root or ⅛ tsp. powdered ginger.
1 tsp. salt
2 tbs. soy sauce
½ cup peanut oil

Slice meat into thin 2 inch pieces (cut against the grain). Stir 1 tbs. oil, 1 tbs. soy sauce into the meat. Cut tomatoes and onions into slices. Heat frying pan and add 3 tbs. of oil. When boiling, put beef in and fry for 3 minutes. Stir constantly. Lower heat and take out meat and place in a bowl. Turn heat high again and add balance of oil and add salt, then stir in onion. Cook for about 2 minutes alone, then add tomatoes. Continue to cook, uncovered, for 10 to 15 minutes at medium heat. Mix ¼ cup water, 1 tbs. soy sauce and the ginger and pour over cooking onions and tomatoes. When sauce is browned, turn off heat and fold meat into tomatoes and onion sauce. Serve at once.

BEEF GOULASH

1½ lbs. chuck steak cubed
2 tbs. oil
4 cups chopped onions

1 tbs. paprika
1 tsp. salt
1 small can tomato paste

Heat oil in heavy saucepan and saute onions until golden brown. Add meat and cook, stirring over medium heat for several minutes. Add all other ingredients and simmer very slowly, covered for about 1½ hours, until tender.

SAMARKAND SOUFFLE

1½ cups millet, cooked (like rice)
½ cup grated cheddar cheese
½ tsp. salt

fresh ground pepper
⅛ tsp. fine herbs
¾ cup milk
3 eggs beaten separately

Mix first 6 ingredients together, reserving half the cheese. Fold in beaten egg whites. Pour into greased casserole. Sprinkle on remainder of cheese. Place casserole in pan of hot water and bake at 350° for about 20 minutes till set. Serves 4

JELLIED CHICKEN SALAD

2 tbs. unflavored gelatin
½ cup cold water
3 cups chicken flavored bouillon
½ cup lemon juice
pinch salt
3 green olives stuffed with pimiento (sliced)
1 cup pineapple tidbits (drained)
2 cups cooked or canned chicken (diced)
½ cup celery chopped
¼ cup green pepper (chopped)

Dissolve gelatin in hot chicken bouillon after softening in cold water. Add lemon juice and salt, and chill. When partially set, pour small amounts of gelatin into individual molds (yield from 8 to 12), place several olive slices in each. Chill until just about set. Stir pineapple, chicken and vegetables into remaining gelatin and pour carefully over gelatin already in molds. Chill until firm and unmold. Serve with mayonnaise.

EGGS EN GELLÉ

½ can beef or chicken consommé
tarragon
1 tbs. unflavored gelatin
eggs

Heat soup and add tarragon and dissolved gelatin. Meanwhile poach eggs. Pour liquid over them in serving bowl and chill.

GEORGIAN CHICKEN

2½ lbs. chicken
7 tbs. clarified butter for frying

14 oz. onions
2½ tbs. flour
3 oz. tomato paste (or 2 oz. or more of fresh tomatoes)
1 tbs. white table wine or vinegar
juice of 1 lemon
greens
spices
salt to taste

Cut up chicken and fry in clarified butter. Transfer to pot, add onion lightly browned in flour and tomato paste (or fresh tomatoes), white wine or vinegar, lemon juice, greens chopped fine and spices. Stew till tender. Serves 4

TOASTED SESAME SEEDS

Preheat oven to 350 degrees. In a baking pan, arrange sesame seeds in a light layer and bake for about 20 minutes until the seeds are a golden brown and have a nut-like flavor. Leftover seeds may be stored in a glass jar that is dry and has a screw cap. For use in salads, creamed dishes and meat loaves.

JELLIED RED CAVIAR

2 tbs. unflavored gelatin
½ cup cold water
16 ozs. tomato juice
grated onion to taste
16 ozs. beef or chicken
    consommé
slice of lemon rind
pinch salt

black pepper
1 tsp. lemon juice
sherry
dash Worcestershire sauce
2 ozs. red caviar
¼ cup sour cream
¼ cup chives (chopped)

Soften gelatin in cold water. Bring to a boil the tomato juice, onion, consommé and lemon rind. Dissolve the gelatin in this hot mixture. Strain and season to taste with salt, pepper, lemon juice, sherry and Worcestershire. Chill in six individual molds until almost set. Stir a teaspoon of caviar into each mold and chill until the soup is set. Before serving, place a tablespoon of sour cream on the top of each mold of soup and sprinkle with chopped chives. Serves 6

CHILLED CANTONESE SHRIMP

2 doz. shrimp, medium sized
(cooked, shelled and deveined, but
with last tail segment left intact)
1 water cress
4 oz. soy sauce
4 oz. lemon juice (freshly squeezed)
1 tsp. ginger

Chill shrimp until ready to serve. Arrange shrimp on a serving dish, garnished with sprigs of water cress. Combine soy sauce, lemon juice and ginger and mix well. Divide mixture evenly into four individual serving dishes to be used as a dip for shrimp and water cress. Serves 4

LUNCHEON SHRIMP

Melt frozen cream of shrimp soup in pan, bring to a boil (no water). Add shrimp and lemon juice.

SWORDFISH (OR SALMON) CURRY

Swordfish cut into 1" cubes
1 tbs. butter
2 tomatoes
½ cucumber
1 tsp. curry powder
⅛ tsp. coriander
pepper and salt to taste
1 cup grated coconut (no water)

Melt 1 tbs. butter in pan. Add cut-up tomatoes, and ½ cut-up cucumber on top. Sprinkle in 1 tsp. curry powder, coriander and pepper and salt. Top with coconut and cook on low flame for 20 minutes.

EAST COAST SKEWERED LAMB

Have 6 lb. leg of lamb cut into 1" cubes
Marinate overnight in refrigerator in sauce made as follows:
Place 2 tbs. cooking oil in saucepan over medium heat; add 1½ tsp. curry powder plus pinch hot red pepper; stir and add 1 cup milk or coconut milk slowly. Then add ½ cup ground peanuts or

¼ cup peanut butter, 2 tbs. good soy sauce plus ¼ tsp. dark molasses, 1 tsp. brown sugar, juice of half a lemon, ⅛ tsp. garlic powder. Cook stirring occasionally for 20 minutes.

Line firebox with quilted aluminum foil. Oil grill. Place lamb cubes on skewers and brown over charcoal about 15 to 20 minutes, turning several times. Serve with chilled crushed pineapple and hot rice. Serves 6

OYSTERS A LA ORIENT

2 doz. oysters	1 tsp. cumin seed
3 tbs. butter	2 red chili peppers (crushed)
½ tbs. parsley (chopped)	yolks of 2 eggs
1 cup sliced mushrooms	4 oz. cream
8 oz. milk	pinch salt
8 oz. buttermilk	

Poach oysters in water and their own liquor. Drain and mince. Add chopped parsley to melted butter and fry for ½ minute before adding mushrooms. Then combine milk and buttermilk and add ⅔ cup at a time, be sure to boil away liquid after each addition. Add the cumin and 2 tbs. water in which crushed peppers have been soaked, discard peppers. Beat the egg yolks with the cream. Add to mushroom mixture with oysters and salt. Cover and remove from heat for 3 minutes before serving. Serves 4

CURRY OF LOBSTER

6 tbs. butter	2 sliced tomatoes
2 onions (sliced)	pinch salt
cinnamon	pinch sugar
powdered cloves	1 tbs. lemon juice
cumin	4 cups milk
chili powder	2 garlic cloves (minced)
1 tsp. coriander	3 lbs. parboiled lobster
1 tbs. turmeric	1 cucumber

Fry sliced onions with cinnamon, cloves, cumin, chili, coriander, turmeric and tomatoes in 3 tbs. melted butter. Mix well and add salt, sugar, lemon juice and milk. Simmer on low heat for 15 minutes. Melt remaining 3 tbs. butter in another pan to lightly fry the garlic. Add lobster and coat it well with butter. Cook for 5 minutes and add the milk and spice sauce. Cook until the liquid is reduced by ⅓. Be sure to keep pan covered. Slice cucumber very thin and add to lobster. Cook altogether for 10 minutes and serve hot. Serves 6

SOUTH AMERICAN SHRIMP

2 lbs. shrimp
¼ cup lemon juice
3 tbs. butter
3 tbs. oil
2 sliced onions
4 tomatoes (chopped)
1 tsp. turmeric
1 tsp. coriander

1 tsp. cumin
½ tsp. mustard seed
2 bay leaves
1 tsp. black pepper
pinch salt
1 pint water
pimientos

In boiling water, place shrimp until pink, and remove. After they are cooled and shelled, wash them in lemon juice and set aside. Melt butter and oil to fry onion, tomatoes, spices, salt and herbs. Simmer in covered pan for 10 minutes over a very low heat. Add shrimp and 1 pint water. Cover and simmer for 30 minutes. Serve with pimento strips arranged on top of shrimp. Serves 4

JAVANESE BARBECUED CHICKEN

2 lbs. chicken that has been
  boned
¾ tsp. vinegar
6 oz. water

½ tsp. cumin
½ tsp. garlic (minced)
pinch salt

On 6" skewers, place the chicken that has been cut into 1½" pieces. Combine the remaining ingredients and dip chicken into this. Cook for about 20 minutes over an open fire. Serve hot with this sauce:
    5 tbs. peanut butter, ½ cup bouillon, 1 tsp. sugar, minced garlic to taste, 1 tsp. soy sauce, 4 oz. milk and dash of paprika, and 1 bay leaf. Serves 3 to 4

SUMMER SALAD

Sprinkle 1 envelope unflavored gelatine on ½ cup cold water to soften. Place over boiling water and stir until thoroughly dissolved. Blend 1 can cream of chicken or cream of mushroom soup with ½ cup cold water, 1 tbs. lemon juice and a dash of black pepper. Add the dissolved gelatine and mix thoroughly. Chill to consistency of unbeaten egg white. Blend in leftover chicken or turkey, diced, ½ cup chopped celery, ¼ cup chopped green pepper, 2 tbs. chopped pimiento and 2 tsp. grated onion with a dash of Worcestershire sauce. Turn into a 3 cup mold or individual molds and chill until firm. Unmold on crisp salad greens and serve with salad dressing. Garnish with radish roses and fresh parsley. Serves 4

BEEF KEBABS

2 lbs. sirloin steak or
    leg of lamb
boiling water
6 tbs. yogurt
1 tsp. ginger
¼ cup minced onion

4 tsp. coriander
2 tsp. turmeric
2 tsp. poppy seed
dash cayenne
2 tsp. salt
¼ cup butter, melted

After cutting meat into 1½ inch pieces, soak in boiling water for 5 minutes and drain. Combine yogurt and seasonings until you form a paste. Coat the meat with this and marinate at least 1 hour. Place on skewers and place under broiler or on a grill for 7 to 10 minutes, until meat is cooked. Be sure to baste well with melted butter while cooking. Serve on skewers. Squares of green pepper, tomato wedges or mushrooms may be broiled with meat and alternated on the skewers, if desired.

CHINESE SHRIMP AND PEPPER

1 large green pepper
¼ cup peanut oil
½ clove garlic, chopped fine
1 tsp. salt
black pepper
1 tsp. ginger
1 lb. shrimp

1½ cups chicken stock
2 tomatoes, quartered
2 tbs. soy sauce
2 tbs. cornstarch
¼ cup cold water
3 scallions, sliced into one inch
    lengths, diagonally

Split pepper in half and discard seeds and white fibers. Cut into strips or one inch squares. In a skillet, heat oil and add garlic, salt, pepper and ginger. Add shrimps immediately and cook for 3 minutes or until the shrimps are red. Be sure to stir frequently. Add green pepper and stir. Add chicken stock and cover while you simmer over moderate heat for 3 to 5 minutes, stirring occasionally. Now add tomatoes and mix well while you cook two or three minutes longer. Combine soy sauce, cornstarch and cold water. Stir into the shrimps and simmer until thickened. Add scallions and heat through and serve immediately. Serves 4

MOUSSE OF HAM & TONGUE

3 tbs. shallots
  (finely chopped)
1 tbs. butter
2 envelopes unflavored gelatin
⅓ cup dry white wine
2 cups hot chicken stock
2 ⅓ cups cooked smoked ham
  (cut into small cubes)
2 tbs. cognac
1½ tbs. tomato paste
pinch salt
black pepper

½ cup cooked tongue
  (finely diced)
1½ tbs. fresh dill
¾ cup whipped heavy cream
salad greens
black and stuffed green olives,
  cut as desired
tomato halves, skinned and
  seeded stuffed with
  cooked peas
cooked tiny carrots

Saute the shallots in butter for 2 to 3 minutes. Soak gelatin in wine. Add chicken stock to gelatin and stir until dissolved. Add shallots. In an electric blender, place ½ cup hot liquid and ⅓ cup ham and blend. Stop motor once and stir down mixture with rubber spatula and finish blending. Pour mixture into bowl and repeat this process until all liquid and ham are blended. Stir in cognac and tomato paste. Add salt and pepper and cool mixture. As mixture starts to thicken, stir in diced tongue, dill and whipped cream. Pack into 1½ quart mold. Chill overnight. Arrange salad greens on plate and unmold the mousse onto greens. Garnish with olives, tomato halves and carrots. Serves 6

This mousse may be served with sour cream and horseradish sauce as follows:
1 cup sour cream
2 tbs. horseradish
1 tsp. mustard

Combine sour cream with horseradish and mustard. Chill until ready to serve. Makes 1 cup

BEEF STROGANOFF

7 tbs. butter
2 tbs. chopped shallots

½ lb. mushrooms, thinly sliced
1 cup sour cream

¾ cup chopped onion
1 tsp. salt
black pepper
2 tsp. paprika
2 cups beef stock
2 lbs. beef tenderloin or bone-
    less sirloin of beef, trim
    all fat and cut into strips
    2x¼x¼

3 tbs. tomato paste
1 tsp. Worcestershire sauce
3 tbs. finely chopped parsley

Heat three tablespoons of the butter in a saucepan and cook the shallots, mushrooms, and onion until it is tender and translucent, but not brown. Stir in paprika and cook until onion is coated. Stir in tomato paste and beef stock. Simmer for 20 minutes, stirring occasionally. Sprinkle meat on both sides with salt and pepper and cook meat on both sides with remaining butter. Be sure to cook meat quickly. Do not overcook. Meat should be rare in the center. Combine sour cream and Worchestershire sauce. Add some of the beef sauce to sour cream mixture. Return to heat and stir. Do not boil. Serve sprinkled with parsley. Serves 6

BURGUNDY HAMBURGERS

1 lb. ground beef
1 tsp. salt
¼ cup Burgundy

freshly ground pepper
1 tbs. minced parsley
1 tbs . minced chives

Combine all ingredients and form in cakes and broil to individual taste. Serves 2 or 3

BROILED SALMON STEAKS

Salmon cut 1" to 2" thick   1 tbs. butter

Brush salmon well with butter and put in a hinged broiler. Grill until fish is brown and the flesh separates easily with a fork and has lost its transparent look.

RAGOUT CHASSEUR

3¼ lbs. lamb, cut into small pieces
Mince 3 medium onions and cook till golden in 2 tbs. butter. Then brown meat on high flame, add large can tomatoes, ½ can Italian tomato paste, 1½ spoon curry powder, one large shot red wine or

white wine, 1½ tsp. rosemary, sprig fresh basil, 2 lbs. mushrooms. Add a few sweet pickles and ½ jar juice (optional).

SAUERBRATEN

Top round—place meat for two days in refrigerator in brine made from pickle brine, Tarragon vinegar, red wine and water, 2 laurel (bay) leaves or peppercorns. Cut slots in meat and insert small pieces of bacon. Melt butter and brown meat and begin to cook on not too high a flame. Baste every 15 to 20 minutes with brine. (4 lbs. meat should take 1½ hours.) Cover pot.

NEAR EAST LAMB

2 lbs. lean lamb (from shoulder, chuck or breast)
2 tsp. salt
pepper to taste
6 tbs. oil
1 cup boiling water
3 medium-sized onions, chopped
1 tbs. flour
2 tsp. curry powder
3 cups hot lamb stock
3 tbs. lemon juice
¼ shredded coconut

Have meat cut into 1" squares and sprinkle with salt and pepper. Saute slowly in 2 tbs. oil in large skillet until slightly brown, turn frequently. Add hot water and simmer for 1 hour in covered skillet. Saute onions in remaining ¼ cup oil until light yellow, stir in flour and brown lightly, add curry powder and then add stock gradually and cook until thickened, stirring constantly. Pour over meat and mix well, cover and simmer about ½ hour or until meat is tender. Add lemon juice and coconut. Serves 6

CHINESE DUCK

1 duck 6-6½ lbs.
½ bunch green onions or scallions

Sauce Ingredients

½ cup soy bean paste
1 oz. fresh ginger root
4 cloves garlic
½ tsp. grated dry orange peel

1 tsp. brown sugar
½ tsp. salt
2 tbs. sherry wine

Preparation: (Sauce)

    A. Mince garlic, ginger and orange peel, add to soy bean paste. Add sugar and sherry. Pound together in a small pot or bowl until they are blended into a smooth paste. Heat with a cup of water added; bring to boiling point. Pour hot sauce into inside of cleaned duck. Sew or skewer opening of duck until tightly closed.

Preparation

    A. Tie duck's neck with string.
    B. Rub soy sauce and honey mixed over entire skin of duck. (Place washed scallions inside duck).
    C. Add sauce as directed to inside of duck, etc.
    D. Preheat oven at 450° for about 5 minutes.
    E. Place duck carefully in uncovered roaster pan; cook until duck is golden brown.
    F. Reduce heat from 450° to 325°. Roast duck forty to fifty minutes at 325°.

How To Serve

Remove strings and skewers. Cut duck in slices with golden brown skin attached to each slice. Pour sauce from duck over meat before serving. Serve remainder of sauce in sauce boat.

LIVER CURRY

4 tbs. butter
3 tbs. onion flakes
1½ cloves garlic, chopped
turmeric
crushed red chili pepper
thyme
black pepper

2 bay leaves
2 lbs. calves or beef liver, cubed
1 ¾ tbs. soy sauce
2 cups milk
1 tomato, chopped

Saute the onions and garlic in melted butter. Stir in the turmeric, red pepper, thyme, black pepper, bay leaves and cook gently for two minutes. Add the liver and sprinkle with soy sauce and fry for four minutes. Add milk, salt and cover. Cook until done, about 15 minutes for calves liver. Stir in tomato to thicken the gravy. Serve hot with fried onion. Serves 4

Vegetables

SPINACH SOUFFLÉ

2 or more cups chopped
    spinach, uncooked
1 chopped onion
1½ cup milk
1 cup cheese
½ cup dry skimmed milk

1½ tsp. salt
dash freshly ground pepper
4 eggs
¼ tsp. basil
1 tsp. Worcester sauce
fresh parsley

Heat 1 cup of milk to simmering. Beat together rest of milk, dry milk, salt and pepper. Add to hot milk and simmer for five minutes, stirring. Let cook a little and add the egg yolks, basil, cheese, chopped parsley and Worcester. Stir well. Add spinach and onion. Fold in stiffly beaten whites and pour into oiled casserole and put into 300° oven for approximately 45 minutes.

STRING BEANS WITH SESAME SAUCE

¾ cup sesame seeds
1 lb. string beans cooked
2 tbs. soy sauce
2 tbs. vinegar

Put seeds in ungreased frying pan and heat for several minutes, stirring constantly until the seeds start to crackle. Place in mortar and crush. Add the soy sauce and vinegar and mix. Stir into cooked string beans and serve.

BROCCOLI SAUTE

Cut off hard parts of stem. Wash and cut into small pieces In skillet place about 2 to 3 tbs. salad oil stirred with half the amount good soy sauce, heat, add broccoli and saute 5 minutes. Add 1 cup water (or vegetable cooking juice) and cook 5 more minutes.

VEGETABLES SAMBAL

Finely chop together

1 tomato
1 small onion
1 garlic clove

Add: ½ tsp. dried ginger.
       grated lemon rind
Fry the above a couple of minutes in oil or butter.
Add 1 cup water
       1 tbs. coconut cream (optional)
Stir until it boils.
Add any cut up vegetable or combination of vegetables such as:
cucumbers, carrots, peppers, onions.

BALI GREEN

Thoroughly wash spinach or broccoli (if broccoli, cut into
pieces). Place in pan with a couple of slices of tomato and red
onion. Slice chili pepper in half, removing seeds. Add 1 tbs. honey.
Fill pot half full of water, add ½ tsp. salt and ¼ tsp. M.S.G. Cover
and cook until tender.

COLE SLAW SALAD (A LA RONDHA)

½ head cabbage finely cut
1 can thawed pineapple (no juice)
1 banana
½ cup sour cream

Into the cabbage and pineapple, slice 1 banana, mix all together with the mayonnaise and sour cream.

SESAME FRUIT SALAD

1 clove garlic (split)   2 navel oranges
½ head lettuce (Boston)   2 tbs. sesame seeds (toasted—
½ head lettuce (Romaine)   see recipe below)
¼ head chicory   ¼ cup citrus-tarragon dressing
1 grapefruit

Rub inside of salad bowl with garlic. Wash lettuce, Romaine
and chicory, pat dry. Break leaves into tiny pieces and place in
salad bowl. Chill. Peel fruits and cut into sections. Remove the
white portion and drain off excess juice. Chill. Arrange fruit sections over greens and sprinkle with sesame seeds. Add dressing,
toss lightly, coating greens thoroughly with dressing. Serves 6 to 8

MUSHROOMS SORENTO

1 lb. mushrooms
3 tbs. oil
1 garlic clove
½ tsp. salt
¼ tsp. pepper
1 tbs. butter
4 anchovy fillets, chopped
2 tbs. chopped parsley
juice of ½ lemon

Slice thinly, thoroughly washed mushrooms. Heat oil in skillet and brown the garlic and remove garlic from skillet. Add mushrooms, salt and pepper and cook over high heat until liquid has evaporated. Add butter, anchovies and parsley and cook over medium heat for five minutes more. Remove from heat and add lemon juice and serve. Serves four

SPICED GREEN BEANS

1 lb. fresh green beans (1" lengths)
¼ cup butter
¼ cup minced onion
½ clove minced garlic
¼ tsp. each of: rosemary, basil
1 tsp. salt

Green beans should be soaked in cold water for 15 minutes. In a 1½ quart saucepan, melt the butter and saute onion, garlic and celery until tender. Add beans, after draining, cook over low heat, covered, for 20 minutes. Add seasonings. Serves 4

PEAS IN LETTUCE

1¼ cup frozen peas (10 oz. pkg.)
2 large lettuce leaves (outside)
pinch salt
1 tbs. butter
½ clove garlic

Break the package of peas into several pieces. In the bottom of a one quart saucepan, place one lettuce leaf. Add peas, salt, butter and garlic and cover with the other lettuce leaf. Cover pan and cook over medium-high heat. Reduce the heat when the lid is hot to the touch and cook for 15 minutes. Remove lettuce and garlic. Serves 4

CELERY AND DILL SEED

celery to make 3 cups chopped
pinch salt
½ tsp. dill seed
1 tbs. butter
½ tsp. pepper

In a one quart saucepan, place the celery that has been rinsed and drained. Cover and cook over medium-high heat. When cover is hot to the touch, reduce heat and cook ten minutes on low flame. Combine celery with remaining ingredients. Serves 4

ZUCCHINI

1 lb. zucchini
1 clove garlic (sliced)
1 tbs. oil
1 tomato (peel and quarter)
1½ tsp. salt
dash orégano
pepper to taste

Clean zucchini by scrubbing with stiff brush. Slice crosswise into thin slices. In oil, saute garlic for one minute in a 1½ quart saucepan. Stir in the zucchini and remaining ingredients. Cover this and cook for fifteen minutes over low heat. Serves 4

HOT SLAW

1 head cabbage
1 tsp. salt
1 tbs. butter
4 oz. milk
½ tsp. carraway seed

Rinse and drain the cabbage and place in a covered pan, about one quart. Place over medium-high heat. Reduce the heat to low when the cover is hot, and cook for five minutes. Add salt, butter, milk and carraway seed and bring to a boil. Serves 4

FRENCH TOMATOES AND GREEN BEANS

2 ripe tomatoes
1 lb. cooked green beans (chilled)
½ cup chopped red onion
½ tsp. salt
pepper
¼ cup wine vinegar
6 oz. oil
½ cup chopped parsley

Wash and dry tomatoes and leave the skins on. Slice the tomatoes. Then take tomatoes and green beans and arrange in separate dishes. Over the tomatoes and beans, sprinkle mixture of onion and salt and pepper. Pour vinegar and oil over the tomatoes and green beans and sprinkle with chopped parsley. Serves 4

Soups

SOUP CREOLE

1 can chicken gumbo soup
1 can clam chowder
2 cans water
¼ cup chopped parsley
2 ozs. bourbon or brandy

Blend soups, water and parsley in a saucepan, heat, stirring occasionally. Before serving, ignite warm bourbon and lower flame into the soup and stir. Serves 4 to 6

SOUP FLAMBÉ

1 can cream of chicken soup
1 can cream of asparagus soup
2 cans water
2 ozs. brandy
chopped nuts

Blend soups and water in a saucepan and heat, stirring occasionally. Before serving, ignite warm brandy and lower flame into the soup and stir. Garnish with chopped nuts. Serves 4 to 6

CHILLED MINT AND CUCUMBER SOUP

3 medium sized cucumbers
3 tbs. butter, unsalted
1 medium sized onion
    chopped fine
white pepper

3 tbs. rice flour
2 tbs. fresh mint, finely
    chopped
10 oz. light cream
4 oz. heavy cream, whipped

Peel cucumbers, saving half of one of them. Finely slice the other 2½ cucumbers and place on plate, sprinkle with salt and let stand for thirty minutes. In a heavy pan, melt butter, add onion and season with salt and pepper. Cook slowly for three minutes, being careful not to brown. Take salted cucumbers and wash in cold water, drain and dry. Add to the onion and cover, cook slowly until cucumbers are soft. Remove from heat, mix in flour and 2 cups of water. Return to heat, stirring until mixture comes to a boil. Then simmer for five minutes. Rub this through a fine strainer. Add mint and chill thoroughly. Blend in the light cream and the whipped cream. Take the ½ cucumber in reserve and shred into the soup. Serves four to six

CAMBODIA CHOWDER

3 lbs. pike
2 doz. shrimp
2 doz. oysters
½ cup butter
4 onions (white) diced
2 bay leaves
crushed red chili pepper
dried orange rind
4 anise seeds

3 ¾ qts. water
1 tbs. turmeric
½ clove garlic, chopped
1 tsp. salt
1 tbs. cashew nuts
4 slices fresh pineapple (or
    canned without juice)
1 tbs. soy sauce

After cleaning fish, cut into small pieces. Clean, shell and wash shrimp. Take oysters out of shells. Brown onions in a pan with melted butter. Add shrimp, bay leaves, red pepper and orange rind (which has been chopped). Over a medium fire, stir for five minutes and add fish with anise seeds. Add one cup water and reduce over a fast fire. Add turmeric, oysters, garlic, salt and 3½ quarts water. Add cashew nuts and boil for one minute before simmering for an additional 15 minutes. Crush pineapple with soy sauce about ten minutes before the dish is ready. Stir the pineapple and soy sauce in and thicken chowder before serving. Serves 6

MULLIGATAWNY SOUP

6 to 8 lbs. chicken backs and
    necks
4 cups water
½ cup sliced carrot
2 tbs. minced onion
½ cup celery, chopped
2 tbs. parsley flakes
½ cup chopped mushroom
    stems

4 tbs. minced onion
¼ cup water
2 tbs. butter
4 tsp. flour
1 tbs. curry powder
4 tsp. salt
½ cup heavy cream

Combine the chicken, water, carrot, onion, celery, parsley flakes and mushroom stems. Cover and cook until chicken is tender, then remove chicken. Soften the 4 tbs. minced onion in ¼ cup water. Brown in 2 tbs. butter. Stir in flour, curry powder and salt. Add chicken stock, gradually and cook for 8 minutes. Put through a fine sieve. Stir in heavy cream. Heat thoroughly but do not boil. If desired, pick a little of the chicken from the bones and add a few pieces to each serving. Serves 6

JELLIED GAZPACHO (Spanish Cold Soup)

1 envelope of gelatin
1½ cups water—divided
1 bouillon cube
⅓ cup vinegar
1 tsp. salt
1 tsp. paprika
½ tsp. basil
¼ tsp. ground cloves

¼ tsp. tabasco
1 clove of garlic—minced
2 tbs. finely chopped onion
½ cup finely chopped green
    pepper
1½ cups finely chopped
    tomatoes
sour cream (optional)

Sprinkle gelatin on ½ cup of water to soften. Place over heat and stir until gelatin is dissolved. Remove from heat, add bouillon cube and stir until dissolved. Add remaining 1 cup of water, vinegar, and seasonings and mix. Chill in refrigerator until of unbeaten egg white consistency. Fold in garlic, chopped peppers, celery, onion, and tomatoes. Cover and chill at least one hour. Turn into soup cups or bowl and garnish with sour cream. Serves 8

Sauces

SAUCE FOR FISH

3 yolks of hard boiled eggs
2 tbs. butter
1 cup white sauce
1 tbs. lemon juice
cayenne pepper

Pound the butter with the yolks of 3 hard boiled eggs. Season with salt and cayenne. Place a cup of white sauce into a saucepan and add lemon juice. Add to sauce and simmer gently. Serve with salmon or sole. Serves 4 or 5.

HOT CAPER SAUCE

3 tsp. chopped capers
1 cup clarified butter
1 tsp. vinegar
1 tsp. anchovy paste
red hot pepper

Heat melted butter sauce and stir in chopped capers and vinegar. Let simmer for a few minutes then add anchovy paste. Add a large pinch of pepper. Serve with broiled salmon. Serves 5 or 6

WHITE FISH SAUCE

6 anchovies (canned)
1 tsp. dry mustard
1 tbs. curry powder
½ clove garlic
½ pint melted butter

3 tsp. capers
4 tbs. sherry
3 tbs. vinegar
¾ cup water

In large mortar, pound garlic, capers and anchovies (boned and skinned). Add spices. Mix thoroughly. Add wine, vinegar and water. Boil for 15 minutes; add melted butter. Reheat and serve. Serves 6

LAMB IN CAPER SAUCE

1 cup clarified butter
1 tbs. chopped capers
2 tsp. vinegar

Heat melted butter sauce and stir capers and vinegar in. Simmer for a few minutes and serve with roast lamb. Serves 5 or 6

HORSERADISH CREAM SAUCE

1¼ cup cream
1 tsp. salt
nutmeg

2 egg yolks
2 tbs. butter
½ cup grated horseradish

Whip the cream, add salt and nutmeg. Beat egg yolks and butter together. Heat, stirring until it thickens. Fold in cream and grated horseradish and simmer. Serve immediately with roast beef. Serves 8

MAYONNAISE SAUCE A LA JAMBON

3 eggs yolks
1 tbs. water
¼ tsp. salt
pinch pepper
pinch cayenne

1 cup olive oil
½ cup vinegar
¼ lb. ham
½ green pepper, chopped
1 tsp. parsley, chopped

Put raw egg yolks in a bowl with water, salt and peppers and beat well. Add oil and vinegar, a little at a time, alternating, while beating, or blend in electric blender. Chop the ham into small pieces, add with chopped green pepper and parsley to the mayonnaise. Excellent with game or cold poultry. Serves 6

BUTTER'N SPICE SAUCE

1 cup flour (substitute by
    blending leftover vege-
    tabes or meat in electric
    blender)
1 tsp. salt

dash pepper
pinch nutmeg
2 or 3 cloves (optional)
2 tbs. butter
1 tbs. vinegar

Season flour (blended vegetable should be same vegetable as that served in the meal, so as not to change the taste of the sauce) with salt, pepper, nutmeg and cloves. Mix to a smooth paste with some water, combine with 1 tbs. butter. Put these ingredients in a

saucepan and let cook slowly for about 15 minutes. (Not necessary to cook if pureed vegetables or meat is used, merely heat.)
Remove from heat and add the remaining butter in small pieces.
Stir constantly so that butter does not rise to surface. Add tablespoon vinegar as the last thing. Serve with cooked vegetables.

TART PARSLEY SAUCE

¼ cup butter
3 egg yolks
1 tbs. chopped parsley
½ tsp. salt

dash pepper
1 tsp. tarragon vinegar
1 tbs. lemon juice

Put butter in top of double boiler, let butter melt slowly, but do
not let it become oily. Beat the egg yolks thoroughly and add to
butter. Stir in lemon juice, season with salt and pepper. Blend all
in well but do not allow to boil because egg yolks will curdle. Add
parsley to the sauce and just before serving add a teaspoon of
tarragon vinegar. The tart flavor compliments the taste of cauliflower or asparagus.

ANCHOVY SAUCE

2 cups clarified butter
juice of ½ small lemon

2 tsp. anchovy paste
pinch hot red pepper

Heat butter, add anchovy, pepper and lemon juice. Serve with
poached salmon. Serves 6

OEUFS AU BEURRE NOIR

4 tbs. clarified butter
4 eggs
1 tbs. vinegar

1 tsp. salt
pinch pepper

Heat butter until dark, but not burned, add seasonings. In skillet, put tablespoon of vinegar, break in 4 eggs carefully and pour
the browned butter over them through a fine strainer. Let cook for
3 minutes. Serve on a warm dish. Serves 2

BROWN BUTTER SAUCE

2 tbs. butter
pinch cayenne pepper
1 tsp. salt

2 tbs. hot vinegar
4 poached eggs
½ tsp. capers

Melt butter in saucepan. Stir until brown. Add salt, pepper and vinegar. Keep very hot and pour over poached eggs. Garnish with capers. Serves 2

EGGS CURRY

2 onions
1 tbs. curry powder
½ pint good vegetable stock

2 tbs. cream
1 tbs. butter
8 hard boiled eggs

Fry thinly sliced onion in butter until colored. Sprinkle with curry powder and blend. Add stock, a little at a time, stirring to keep smooth. Cook for 15 minutes. Then add cream, a little at a time, stirring constantly. Slice hard-boiled eggs. Heat in the sauce until hot. Serve at once. Serves 4 to 5

HERB BUTTER

¼ lb. butter
2 tbs. minced parsley
¼ tbs. minced chives

1 tsp. lemon juice
1 tsp. minced tarragon

Cream butter with rest of the ingredients.

Slenderizing Snacks

SNACK TRAY & DIP

Celery filled with cottage cheese and sprinkled with paprika, raw cauliflower broken into flowerettes, carrot sticks, scallions, radishes, celery cut into strips. In the center place the following dip:

1 cup mayonnaise (see recipe below)
3 tbs. horseradish mustard
3 tsp. Worcester sauce
1 tsp. grated horseradish

Mix all ingredients together thoroughly and keep refrigerated until used.

HOME-MADE MAYONNAISE

1 egg yolk
1 scant tsp. honey
2 tbs. vinegar or lemon juice
½ tsp. salt

1 tsp. dry mustard or ginger
dash freshly ground pepper
⅛ tsp. paprika
⅛ tsp. basil or tarragon

1 cup soy oil or olive oil or half and half

Can be made in blender or in electric mixer. In blender, blend all ingredients briefly, reserving the oil. Add oil slowly until just mixed. Refrigerate. In a mixer add half the vingear and remaining ingredients, then the oil, first drop by drop and then in an increasing stream, beating as it thickens. Then add remaining vinegar and beat a little more.

Desserts

PINEAPPLE CHIFFON

1½ cups canned crushed pineapple without syrup
2 tbs. plain gelatin
3 eggs separated
½ cup ice-water
½ cup dry skimmed milk
1 tbs. lemon juice
¼ tsp. salt

Stir gelatin and salt together in pan. Add the slightly beaten egg yolks; stir in the pineapple and cook over boiling water or on low heat until gelatin dissolves. Remove from heat, add lemon juice and chill until slightly thickened. Fold into mixture 3 stiffly beaten egg whites. In blender or electric mixer beat water and dry milk until stiff. Fold into gelatin mixture. Spoon one-quarter of mixture into loaf pan, repeat two or more times and finish with the mixture. Chill for 3-4 hours.

APPLE SNOW

2 tbs. gelatin
¼ tsp. salt
¾ cup water
½ tsp. grated lemon rind

1 tbs. lemon juice
1 lb. can sugar-free apple-
    sauce (1¾ cup)
2 egg whites, unbeaten

In pan mix together gelatin and salt. Add water and cook stirring over low heat or over boiling water until dissolved. Remove from heat and add lemon rind, lemon juice and applesauce. Chill until slightly thickened. Add the egg white to mixture and beat in electric mixer or blender until it begins to be firm. Spoon into one large mold or individual molds or glasses. Chill.

ARUBA WHIP

Whip white of 1 egg till stiff. Add to it cut-up ripe avocado. Mix together. Add 1½ tbs. lemon juice and 1½ tbs. honey. Beat all together. Put into wine glasses and top with whipped cream. Serves 4

FOUR FRUITS IN KIRSCH

Place four fruits, including melon, cut into small pieces and strawberries, sliced or mashed, in compote dish. Sprinkle with two tablespoons chopped nuts and drizzle Kirsch over it all. Chill.

PEACH PARFAIT

2 baby jars peaches
½ pt. whipped cream

Fill 4 parfait glasses with alternate peaches and whipped cream. Top with a little creme de menthe.

COFFEE CUSTARD

1 cup milk scalded
1 cup strong coffee
4 tbs. sugar (brown)

⅛ tsp. salt
¾ tsp. vanilla
dash of mace

Mix coffee and milk and scald. Blend together the rest of ingredients and add to scalded milk. Place baking dish in pan of hot water and cook in slow oven (325°) until set. Serves 4

CHIFFON CREME

1 tbs. gelatin
¼ cup cold water
¼ cup boiling water

4 tbs. brown sugar
1 cup cream, whipped
1 tsp. vanilla

Blend gelatin into cold water. Cook stirring with boiling water until dissolved. Add sugar and stir thoroughly. Remove from heat and chill. When beginning to set, fold in whipped cream flavored with vanilla. Spoon into sherbert cups and chill until set.

ZABAGLIONE

4 egg yolks
4 tbs. honey
4 tbs. dry red wine

Place ingredients over medium direct heat and bring to gentle boil, beating constantly until thick and fluffy. Place in sherbert glasses. May be served warm or cold. Serves 4

CREME DE MOCHA

2 broken-up bars sweet
    chocolate
2 tbs. instant coffee
1 tbs. honey

1 cup cream, ½ whipped
4 beaten egg yolks
1 tsp. vanilla
sprinkle mace or cinnamon

Mix together chocolate, coffee, honey and ½ the unwhipped cream until smooth, stirring over medium heat. Add egg yolk and continue cooking and stirring for a few minutes. Remove from heat and add vanilla. Pour into sherbet glasses and garnish with rest of whipped cream.

MOUSSE AU CHOCOLAT

1 egg white beaten till stiff
½ pt. cream, whipped

½ package chocolate bits
dash nutmeg

Melt chocolate bits until almost completely dissolved; add immediately to combined whipped cream and beaten egg white. Add nutmeg and refrigerate. Serves 4

BAVARIAN CREME AU CAFE

1 tbs. unflavored gelatin
¾ cup black coffee
2 eggs
½ cup sugar or equivalent artificial sweetening
½ cup milk

¾ tsp. vanilla
1 cup heavy cream, whipped

While the gelatine is softening in ½ the coffee, make a custard of the beaten egg yolks, half the sweetening. Add milk slowly. Cook over medium heat, stirring constantly. When it is slightly thickened, add the softened gelatin and stir. Remove from heat, add vanilla and the rest of the coffee and refrigerate until thickened. Meanwhile beat egg-whites until stiff, gradually adding rest of the sweetening. Fold whipped cream and egg whites into chilled mixture. Can be piled into sherbet glasses or into a one-quart mold. Chill until serving time.

MOCHA SPONGE

8 squares bitter-sweet baking chocolate
2 tbs. butter
½ cup evaporated milk
4 eggs separated
1 envelope unflavored gelatin
¼ cup black coffee
⅓ cup cream, whipped

Melt chocolate and butter in milk over medium heat, stirring. Cool slightly and stir in egg yolks which have been beaten. Cook, stirring till slightly thickened, over low flame. Soften gelatin in coffee and add to hot mixture. Continue stirring for about 1 minute. Remove from heat. Fold in stiffly beaten egg whites and chill. Top with whipped cream.

FRAISES DU BOIS

In blender, place strawberries, a touch of Kirsh, honey to taste and a little heavy cream. Blend together. Place in bowl and decorate with fresh strawberries and chill.

TABLE OF
CARBOHYDRATE (CARBO-CAL) CONTENT
OF COMMON FOODS AND DRINKS

Each food or drink is identified with a symbol as follows:

O This is a GO food—few carbo-cals or none. Can be eaten in abundance without endangering your weight program.

□ This food contains a moderate amount of carbo-cals, but use CAUTION in including this type of food in your diet for maximum weight control purposes.

+ This is classified as a STOP food because it is heavy in carbo-cals. STOP foods are detrimental to your program of weight control.

Alcoholic Beverages

ITEM	PORTION	CARBO-CALS	CALORIES
Ale +			
Domestic +	8 oz. beer	32	150
Imported +	8 oz. beer	40	160
Alexander, Brandy □	3 oz. cocktail	12	185
Alexander, Gin □	3 oz. cocktail	12	180
Anisette +	1 oz. cordial	28	80
Apple Jack O	1 oz. pony	2	100
Bacardi Cocktail □	3 oz. cocktail	14	100

ITEM	PORTION	CARBO-CALS	CALORIES
B & B ☐	1 oz. pony	7	80
Beer, Bock +	8 oz. beer	35	175
Beer, Half and Half +	8 oz. beer	30	135
Beer, Lager +	8 oz. beer	30	125
Benedictine +	1 oz. cordial	26	80
Bloody Mary ☐	6 oz.	20	150
Bourbon & Soda (Highball) ○	8 oz.	0	100
Bourbon & Ginger (Highball) +	8 oz.	65	250
Bourbon ○	1½ oz.	0	100
Brandy, Apricot ○	1 oz. cordial	0	75
Brandy, California ○	1 oz. cordial	0	70
Brandy Cocktail ○	3 oz. cordial	0	70
Brandy, Imported ○	1 oz. cordial	0	75
Brandy Sour +	6 oz. delmonico	24	155
Brandy Toddy +	6 oz. oldfashioned	20	140
Bronx Cocktail ☐	3 oz. cordial	15	105
Buttered Rum (Hot Toddy) ○	8 oz. T & J Mug	0	350
Canadian Whiskey ○	1 oz. pony	0	100
	1½ oz.	0	150
Chablis ○	4 oz. wine	2	140
Champagne domestic ☐	4 oz.	12	100
French ○	4 oz.	4	80
Champagne Cocktail +	4 oz.	36	175
Chartreuse +	1 oz. cordial	26	85
Cherry Heering +	1 oz. cordial	24	100
Cider (Fermented) ☐	6 oz.	7	50
Claret Wine ○	4 oz. wine	2	125
Cognac ○	1 oz. pony	0	75
Creme de Cocoa +	1 oz. cordial	24	95
Creme de Menthe +	1 oz. cocktail	24	90
Creme de Menthe Frappe +	3 oz. cocktail	28	120
Cuba Libre +	10 oz. Tom Collins	40	205
Curacao +	1 oz.	24	100
Daiquiri +	3 oz. cocktail	2C	180
Dubonnet +	3 oz. cocktail	48	155
French '75 +	8 oz. highball	38	280

ITEM	PORTION	CARBO-CALS	CALORIES
Gin ◯	1½ oz. jigger	0	112
	1 oz. pony	0	75
Gin Buck +	10 oz. highball	30	165
Gin Collins +	10 oz. Tom Collins	24	155
Gin Fizz +	10 oz. highball	28	165
Gin Rickey □	10 oz. highball	6	140
Grasshopper +	3 oz. cocktail	72	235
Horse's Neck +	10 oz. Tom Collins	36	190
Irish Coffee +	6 oz.	22	80
Irish Whiskey ◯	1 oz. pony	0	100
	1½ oz.	0	150
Jack Rose +	3 oz. cocktail	18	145
Kummel +	3 oz. cocktail	24	80
Madeira +	3½ oz.	18	120
Manhattan +	3 oz. cocktail	32	260
Martini (Dry) ◯	3 oz. cocktail	1	200
Martini (Sweet) +	3 oz. cocktail	32	190
Mint Julep □	10 oz. Tom Collins	12	355
Muscatel +	3½ oz.	56	170
Old Fashioned +	3 oz.	30	175
Orange Blossom +	3 oz. cocktail	16	165
Pink Lady □	3 oz. cocktail	12	170
Planter's Punch +	10 oz. Tom Collins	32	365
Port +	4 oz. wine	68	135
	3½ oz.	56	110
Porter or Stout +	8 oz.	40	200
Riessling □	4 oz. wine	8	135
Rhine Wine □	4 oz. wine	8	150
Rob Roy	3 oz. cocktail		
w/dry vermouth ◯		1	110
regular +		32	230
Rum Collins +	10 oz. Tom Collins	36	175
Rum Fizz +	8 oz. highball	28	125
Rum & Cola +	8 oz. highball	80	260
Rum Jamaica ◯	1 oz. pony	0	100
Rum Bacardi ◯		0	60
Rum Punch +	8 oz. punch cup	32	300
Rye Highball	8 oz. highball		
w/soda ◯		0	100
w/ginger ale +		64	200

ITEM	PORTION	CARBO-CALS	CALORIES
Rye Whiskey ○	1 oz. pony	0	100
	1½ oz.	0	150
Sautern (sweet) +	4 oz. wine	20	95
	3½ oz.	16	80
Sazerac ☐	3 oz. cocktail	10	180
Scotch Manhattan +	6 oz. oldfashioned	0	85
Scotch Mist ○	3 oz. cocktail	32	235
Scotch & Soda ○	8 oz. highball	0	90
Scotch Whiskey ○	1 oz. pony	0	85
	1½ oz.	0	130
Screwdriver +	8 oz.	60	250
Sherry +	2½ oz. sherry	14	95
	3½ oz.	20	130
Sidecar +	3 oz. cocktail	18	150
Singapore Sling +	8 oz. highball	60	175
Sloe Gin ○	1 oz. pony	0	55
	1½ oz. jigger	0	85
Sloe Gin Collins +	10 oz. Tom Collins	30	170
Sloe Gin Fizz +	8 oz. highball	15	155
Sloe Gin Rickey +	10 oz. highball	25	150
Stinger +	3 oz. cocktail	36	185
Stout +	8 oz. beer	50	140
Tom Collins +	10 oz. Tom Collins	36	155
Tom & Jerry +	8 oz. T & J mug	60	335
Vermouth (Dry or French) ○	4 oz. wine	5	105
	3½ oz.	4	92
Vermouth (Sweet or Italian) +	4 oz. wine	55	175
	3½ oz.	48	153
Vodka ○	1½ oz. jigger	0	180
Ward Eight +	8 oz. stem	30	230
Whiskey Fizz +	8 oz. highball	20	160
Whiskey Highball (Soda) ○	8 oz. highball	0	175
Whiskey Sour +	3 oz. cocktail	16	200
Wine, Dry Red ○ (Chiante, Claret, Burgundy)	3½ oz.	2	70
Wine, Sour ○	3½ oz. (Dry)	2	95

ITEM	PORTION	CARBO-CALS	CALORIES
Wine, Sweet +	4 oz. wine	40	130
Wine, Dry White ○	3½ oz.	2	75
(Chablis, Moselli, Rhine)			
Zinfandel □	4 oz. wine	10	85
Zombi +	14 oz.	100	500

Beverages

ITEM	PORTION	CARBO-CALS	CALORIES
Apple Juice +	1 cup canned	120	124
	1 cup fresh	120	123
Apricot Juice, +	1 cup	120	175
unsweetened	4 oz. glass	60	80
Apricot Nectar +	1 cup	144	160
Blackberry Juice +	1 cup	80	70
	4 oz. glass	40	35
Blueberry Juice +	4 oz. glass	56	130
Carbonated Soda +			
(Sweet)	8 oz.	80	105
Carbonated Water,			
Seltzer ○	8 oz.	0	5
Carrot Juice +	1 cup	50	50
	4 oz. glass	25	25
Cherry Soda +	8 oz.	80	80
Chocolate Beverage +			
(w/milk)	1 cup	68	140
Cider, Apple			
(sweet) +	8 oz.	100	115
Clam Juice □	4 oz. glass	8	45
Cocoanut Milk □	8 oz. glass	8	60
Coffee ○	8 oz.	0	0
Cola Type			
Beverages +	8 oz.	100	105
Cranberry Juice +	1 cup	140	140
Cream Soda +	8 oz.	100	105
Currant Juice +			
Black	1 cup	136	140
Red	1 cup	100	110
Egg & Fruit Punch +	8 oz.	110	275
Eggnog +	8 oz.	100	270
(All milk & one egg)			

ITEM	PORTION	CARBO-CALS	CALORIES
Fruit Punch +	8 oz. glass	170	200
Ginger Ale			
(Pale Ale) +	8 oz.	84	100
Grapefruit Juice +	1 cup	82	87
canned,			
unsweetened +	1 cup	90	92
canned,			
sweetened +	1 cup	120	131
frozen,			
unsweetened +	6 oz. can	288	297
frozen,			
unsweetened,			
diluted +	1 cup	96	105
frozen,			
sweetened +	6 oz. can	320	340
frozen,			
sweetened,			
diluted +	1 cup	112	125
Grape Juice +	1 cup	172	180
frozen, sweet +	1 cup	128	130
undiluted +	4 oz. glass	80	85
Grape Soda +	8 oz.	90	100
Grapefruit-Orange +			
canned,			
sweetened +	8 oz. glass	125	131
canned,			
sweetened +	3 fl. oz.	48	52
canned,			
unsweetened +	8 oz. glass	90	99
canned,			
unsweetened ☐	3 fl. oz.	35	40
frozen,			
condensed +	1 can-6 fl. oz.	280	297
frozen,			
condensed,			
diluted 1—3 ☐	3 fl. oz.	38	42
frozen, condensed,			
undiluted ☐	3 fl. oz.	130	149
Kaffee Hag ○	8 oz.	0	0
Lemonade, diluted +	1 cup	112	120

ITEM	PORTION	CARBO-CALS	CALORIES
Lemon Juice ○	1 cup	80	80
	1 tbs.	5	5
Lemon Soda +	8 oz.	112	115
Lime Juice □	1 cup	40	48
	4 oz.	20	24
Limeade +			
frozen,			
concentrated +	6 oz. can	400	420
frozen, diluted +	1 cup	108	120
Low Calorie,			
Most Flavors ○	8 oz.	0	2
Orange Juice +			
concentrated,			
canned +	1 tbs.	14	16
concentrated, frozen,			
undiluted +	1 tbs.	10	10
concentrated, frozen,			
undiluted +	6 oz. can	320	330
Dehydrated +	4 oz. crystals	400	400
Dehydrated, water			
added +	1 cup	108	110
Canned,			
sweetened +	8 oz.	140	140
Canned,			
unsweetened +	8 oz.	112	115
Fresh +	8 oz.	100	108
California			
Valencia +	1 cup	104	108
Florida			
Early Season +	1 cup	92	100
Florida			
Late Season +	1 cup	104	108
Orange Soda +	8 oz.	92	95
Orangeade +	8 oz.	70	100
Nectarine Juice +	1 cup	140	150
Papaya Juice Ade +	8 oz.	120	120
Papaya, Plain □	4 oz.	50	65
Peach Nectar,			
canned +	1 cup	112	116
	4 oz.	64	65
Pear Nectar,	1 cup	120	125

ITEM	PORTION	CALS CARBO-	CALORIES
canned +	4 oz.	60	60
Pepsi Cola +	8 oz.	108	120
Pineapple Juice-Ade +	8 oz.	90	95
Pineapple Juice, canned +	½ cup	60	60
Frozen, sweetened +	½ cup	60	97
Pomegranate Juice +	4 oz.	60	75
Postum, Black ○	8 oz.	0	0
Prune Juice, canned +	4 oz.	80	85
Quinine Water □	8 oz.	36	40
Raspberry Juice +	4 oz.	60	66
Root Beer +	8 oz.	98	100
Sarsaparilla +	8 oz.	98	100
Sauerkraut Juice □	4 oz.	16	25
Seltzer, See Carbonated Water			
Tangerine Juice, Canned +	1 cup	108	110
canned, unsweetened +	1 cup	100	110
frozen, diluted +	1 cup	108	120
frozen, undiluted +	6 oz. can	320	330
fresh +	4 oz.	40	48 .
Tea ○	8 oz.	0	0
w/lemon ○	8 oz.	1	2
See Chart for Milk & Sugar			
Tomato Juice □	1 cup	40	50
	4 oz.	20	25
Vegetable Juice □	1 cup	36	50
	4 oz.	18	25
V-8 Juice □	1 cup	36	50
	4 oz.	18	25

Breads

Bagel +	1 med. size	120	125
Baking Powder	2½" diameter	80	130
Biscuits +	1 small	56	90

ITEM	PORTION	CARBO-CALS	CALORIES
Banana Bread +	1 slice	88	100
Blueberry Muffin +	2½" diameter	92	100
Boston Brown Bread +	slice-¾"	84	86
Unenriched flour +	slice	90	105
Degermed flour +	slice	86	100
Bran Bread +	slice	68	75
w/raisins +	slice	108	120
Bran Muffins +	3½" diameter	80	85
Bread Crumbs, dry +	½ cup	120	170
Brown Nut Bread +	slice	96	100
Cinnamon Buns +	2½" sq.	100	140
w/raisins +	1	112	155
Cinnamon Bread +	1 slice	94	135
Cinnamon Toast +	1 slice	90	130
Clover Leaf Roll +	1	80	150
Corn Muffins +	1	72	105
Cornmeal Muffins +	2-¾" diameter	80	135
Corn Bread +	1 qu. pc.	70	105
Date Muffins +	2-¾" diameter	130	140
Date & Nut +	slice	102	105
Egg Muffins +	2½" diameter	80	85
English Muffin,			
toasted +	1	120	125
Frankfurter Roll +	1	40	160
French Bread +	1 sm. slice	42	70
French Roll, Hard +	3½" diameter	65	100
French Toast Without			
syrup +	1 pc.	56	130
w/1 tbs. corn			
syrup +	1 pc.	120	250
w/1 tbs. maple			
syrup +	1 pc.	125	260
Gingerbread +	1 square	40	180
Gluten Bread +	slice	32	35
Graham +	slice	44	75
Hamburger Roll +	1 reg.	80	155
Hard Roll +	1	100	155
Hot Cross Bun +	1	80	180
Italian +	1 sm. slice	40	50

ITEM	PORTION	CARBO-CALS	CALORIES
Melba Toast +	slice	32	40
Pecan Buns +	1	108	150
Petit Fours +	1	100	180
Plain Muffins +	2-¾" diameter	64	135
Onion Roll +	4" diameter	120	150
Parkerhouse Roll +	1	75	125
Plain Biscuits or Buns +	1	80	125
w/enriched flour +	1	85	135
Popover +	1	10	60
Protein +	slice	36	60
Pumpernickel +	slice	60	75
Raisin +	slice	70	80
Raisin Muffins +	1 regular	108	130
Roman Meal +	1 slice	52	80
Rye +			
light +	1 slice	60	75
dark +	1 slice	56	70
Party Sliced +	1 slice	32	40
Rye & Wheat +	1 slice	56	70
Soya +	1 slice	35	65
Soy Muffins +	1 medium	64	80
Spoon Bread +	1 serving	68	110
Swedish Health Bread +	2" square	30	50
Sweet Rolls +	3½" diameter	84	135
Vienna +	1 sm. slice	40	55
White, slice +	1 slice	48	64
White, plain Muffin +	1 medium	68	135
Cracked Wheat +	slice	48	80
Whole Wheat +	slice	44	55
Whole Wheat Muffin +	1 medium	68	130
Whole Wheat Roll +	1 medium	68	90
Zweibach +	1 pc.	20	25

Cakes

Almond +	1 pc.	128	175
Angel Food +	1/12 of 8" diameter	100	110
Apple Crumb +	1 med. pc.	200	220
Applesauce +	1 med. pc.	75	150

ITEM	PORTION	CARBO-CALS	CALORIES
Butter Cake +	1 med. pc.	144	200
w/icing +		180	250
Caramel, with icing +	1 med. pc.	170	210
without icing +	1 med. pc.	140	175
Cheese cake +	1 med. pc.	120	300
Cheese cake with pineapple +	1 med. pc.	160	310
Chocolate Layer no icing +	1 med. pc.	56	100
with icing +	1 sm. pc.	70	155
no icing +	1 lg. pc.	88	150
with icing +	1 lg. pc.	180	190
Chocolate Loaf +	1 med. pc.	130	150
Chocolate Eclair, cream +	1 med. pc.	120	300
Chocolate Eclair, custard +	1 med. pc.	110	250
Cocoanut +	3" wedge	200	250
Coffee +	1 med. pc.	105	150
Plain +	1 med. pc.	120	130
iced with nuts +	1 med. pc.	135	150
Cupcake +	1 med. circular	75	161
with icing +		120	180
Date Torte +	1 serving	110	180
Devil's Food +	1 med. pc.	140	150
Doughnuts +			
french +	1 med. cruller	80	140
iced +	1 med. solid	95	250
iced +	1 med. with hole	90	220
Jelly +	1 med. size	120	230
Jelly +	1 sm. size	110	210
Plain cake +	1 med. size	68	162
Plain cake +	1 med. size with hole	52	136
Sugar +	1 med. with hole	84	196
Twist +	1 med. size	80	191
Foundation +	1 med. pc.	120	230
Fruit +	2"x2"x½" pc.	88	105
Ginger +	1 med. pc.	100	110
Gold +	1 med. pc.	60	180
Ice Box +	1 med. pc.	110	235
Jelly Roll +	1 slice	135	150

ITEM	PORTION	CARBO-CALS	CALORIES
Layer, 2 with icing +	1 med. pc.	90	100
3 with icing +	1 med. pc.	120	225
round with icing +	1/6 of 6" diameter	130	241
round with icing +	1/16 of 10" diameter	190	322
Marble +	1 slice	120	200
Nut Loaf +	1 slice	100	110
Orange Cupcake +	1 pc.	80	190
Pancakes, buckwheat +	4" diameter	40	47
enriched flour +	4" diameter	50	60
wheat +	4" diameter	50	59
Pineapple Upsidedown +	1 pc.	280	300
Plain Cake +	1 pc.	120	160
Popovers +	3" diameter	50	60
Potato Cake +	3" arc	100	180
Pound +	1 med. pc.	72	130
Rich Cake, no icing +	1 med. pc. square	200	294
icing +	1 med. pc. round		
	1/16 of 6" diameter	250	378
Short Cakes, plain +	1 med. square	100	142
Strawberry +	1 med. square	240	320
Peach +	small portion	160	185
Raspberry +	med. portion	200	240
Strawberry Sponge +	med. portion	240	260
Spice Cake +	2" cube	108	180
Sponge Cake +	1/12 of 8" diameter	84	117
Sunshine +	1 med. square	144	180
Vanilla, no icing +	1 med. pc.	60	100
with icing +	1 sm. pc.	70	100
Washington			
Cream Cake +	3½" wedge	160	200
White Cake +	2" square	96	155

Cereals

ITEM	PORTION	CARBO-CALS	CALORIES
All Bran +	8 oz. cup	168	180
	½ cup	84	90
Barley +	1 tbs.	40	50
Bran Flakes,			
40% Bran +	8 oz. cup	100	115
Bran, Raisin +	8 oz. cup	120	149

ITEM	PORTION	CARBO-CALS	CALORIES
Bran, Whole Cereal +	8 oz. cup	40	240
Cheerios +	8 oz. cup	68	98
Corn Flakes +	8 oz. cup	84	95
Cream of Wheat, cooked +	8 oz. cup	100	110
Farina, cooked +	8 oz. cup	52	120
Force +	8 oz. cup	60	180
Grapenuts +	8 oz. cup	320	400
Grapenuts Flakes +	¾ cup	72	220
Infants, Dry, precooked +	1 oz.	80	100
K Cereal +	1 serving	48	105
Kellogg's Concentrate +	½ cup	28	100
Kix Cereal +	8 oz. cup	80	128
Krispies +	8 oz. cup	120	136
Krumbles +	8 oz. cup	110	142
Maypo, Coat Cooked +	¾ cup	84	140
Oat Cereal, Ready-to-Eat +	8 oz. cup	68	100
Oatmeal, Infant Dry, precooked +	1 oz. portion	60	106
Oatmeal, Cooked +	8 oz. cup	104	148
Dry, Rolled Oats +	8 oz. cup	85	312
Pablum Cereal +	½ cup - 4 oz.	50	90
Pep Cereal +	8 oz. cup	90	125
Post Toasties +	8 oz. cup	80	110
Puffed Corn +	¾ cup	100	120
Puffed Rice +	8 oz. cup	46	55
Puffed Wheat +	8 oz. cup	40	55
Sweetened +	1 oz.	68	80
Ralston Health Cereal +	8 oz. cup	120	200
Ralston, Hot or Instant uncooked +	½ cup	80	95
Ralston Wheat Chex +	½ cup	90	120
Rice Flakes +	8 oz. cup	108	120
Rice Krispies +	8 oz. cup	100	125
Rolled Oatmeal, cooked +	8 oz. cup	110	148
Rolled Oatmeal, infant, dry, precooked +	1 oz. portion	90	106

ITEM	PORTION	CARBO-CALS	CALORIES
Rolled Oats, Cereal			
(Ready-to-Eat) +	8 oz. cup	80	100
Roman Meal +	½ cup	100	135
Rye Flakes +	8 oz. cup	75	125
Scotch Oatmeal,			
cooked +	8 oz. cup	118	150
Shredded Wheat,			
Biscuit +	1 oz. piece	72	100
Sugar Krisp +	1 cup	104	160
Wheat Flakes +	8 oz. cup	92	125
Wheat Germ +	2 tbs.	40	78
Wheat Meal, cereal +	8 oz. cup	118	175
Wheat & Malted Barley,			
cooked +	¾ cup	85	110
Wheatena, cooked +	⅔ cup	80	105
Wheaties, cereal +	8 oz. cup	92	125
Whole Meal, cooked +	8 oz. cup	160	175
Whole Meal, cooked			
w/wheat germ +	8 oz. cup	90	133

Cheeses

ITEM	PORTION	CARBO-CALS	CALORIES
American Cheese ○	1 slice/1 oz.	trace	100
Dry and grated ○	1 tbs.	trace	35
Fresh and grated ○	1 tbs.	trace	35
Blue Cheese ○	1 tbs.	trace	52
	1 oz.	trace	100
Domestic ○	1 oz.	trace	100
Brie ○	1 square pc.	trace	100
	1 oz.	trace	100
Camembert Cheese ○	1 triangle/1 oz.	trace	85
Chateau Cheese ○	1 oz. pc.	trace	100
Cheddar Cheese ○	1" cube/1 oz.	trace	113
Processed ○	1" cube/1 oz.	trace	105
Cottage Cheese □	8 oz. cup	16	240
	1 oz.	2	30
Creamed □	8 oz. cup	24	230
Cream Cheese ○	1 oz.	trace	106
	1 tbs.	trace	56
Edam Cheese ○	1 oz.	trace	120

ITEM	PORTION	CARBO-CALS	CALORIES
Farmer Cheese ○	4 oz. pc.	trace	155
Garganzola Cheese ○	1 oz. pc.	trace	100
Grated Cheese, Dry ○	1 tbs.	trace	35
Grated Cheese, Fresh ○	1 tbs.	trace	30
Liederkranz Cheese ○	2 tbs.	trace	100
Limburger Cheese ○	2 tbs.	trace	97
Mysost +	1 oz.	60	130
Neufchatel Cheese ○	1 tbs.	trace	50
Pabst-ett ○	1 oz.	8	100
Parmesan Cheese ○	1 slice/1 oz.	trace	100
Fresh Grated ○	1 tbs.	trace	35
Dry Grated ○	1 tbs.	trace	30
Pot Cheese ○	1 tbs.	trace	25
	4 oz.	trace	55
Provolone Cheese ○	2 tbs.	trace	98
Roquefort Cheese ○	1" sq./1 oz.	trace	87
Cream Spread ○	2 tbs.	trace	102
Cheese Souffle ☐	½ cup	20	280
Cheese Spreads ☐			
Bacon ☐	1 oz.	8	
Old English Cheese Spread ☐	2 tbs.	8	100
Olive Pimento Spread ☐	2 tbs.	8	87
Pimento Spread ☐	2 tbs.	8	102
	1 oz	8	100
Pineapple Spread ☐	1 oz	8	100
Relish Spread ☐	1 oz	8	100
Roka Spread ☐	1 oz	8	100
Swiss Cheese, Processed ○	1 slice/1 oz	trace	101
	1 slice/1 oz.	trace	105
Gruyere Cheese ○	1 slice/1 oz.	trace	98
Velveeta ☐	1 oz.	12	100
Welsh Rarebit +	1 slice and 4 tbs.	88	200

Cookies

Animal Crackers +	6 pcs.	36	48
Arrowroot +	1	14	50

ITEM	PORTION	CARBO-CALS	CALORIES
Boston +	1	10	25
Brownies +	1 med. sq.	64	135
Butter +	1	28	42
Butterscotch +	1	56	90
Chocolate +	½" diameter	24	50
Chocolate Chip +	2" diameter	32	40
Chocolate Marshmallow +	1	32	80
Cocoanut Bar +	1	40	90
Date Bar +	1	68	104
Devils Food Square +	1	44	80
Fig Newton +	1 lg.	44	87
Gaiety Creme Sandwich +	1	56	110
Chocolate +	1	60	130
Ginger Snaps +	3" diameter	40	50
Graham Crackers +	3½" square	20	25
Chocolate Covered +	2½" square	28	45
Hermit +	1	28	35
Honey +	1	28	50
Lady Fingers +	1 average	36	40
Lorna Doones +	1	20	35
Macaroons, Almond +	1	40	50
Cocoanut +	1	50	55
Marshmallow +	3	136	224
Mollasses +	1	20	25
Nabisco +	4	30	50
Oatmeal +	1	48	84
Oatmeal Wafers +	1	40	60
Oreo +	1	30	52
Orange Thins +	1	32	50
Peanut +	1	28	55
Petit Fours +	1 average	58	150
Plain & Assorted +	1 average	28	109
Raisin +	1	50	110
Sandwich Type +			
Scotch Short Bread +	1 average square	20	35
Short Bread +	1 sq.	20	40
Social Tea +	1 average	16	22
Sour Cream +	1	36	60
Sugar +	1	28	45

ITEM	PORTION	CARBO-CALS	CALORIES
Sugar Wafers +	1	44	80
Tea, Oriental +	1	16	20
Vanilla +	1	12	31
Vanilla Wafers +	1	16	38
Waffle Creams +	1	28	50
Walnut +	1	64	140
Wafers, Assorted +	1	30	44

Crackers

ITEM	PORTION	CARBO-CALS	CALORIES
Animal Crackers +	1	6	8
Butter Crackers +	1	12	20
Cheese Tidbits +	15 tiny	12	20
Croutons, toasted +	½" cube	2	5
Matzoth +	1-4x8 in. sq.	30	50
	1-6" pc.	120	150
Melba +	1	16	20
Oyster +	10 sm. pcs.	28	43
Peanut-Butter-Cheese Sandwich +	1	20	40
Pilot +	1	72	96
Pretzels +	3 pcs.	10	50
Sticks +	7 pcs.	7	8
Ritz Crackers +	1	8	12
Rusk, Holland +	1	34	50
Saltines +	1 square	12	18
Soda +	1 medium	18	24
Soy Bean +	¼ cup	2	70
Swedish Health Bread +	1 square	40	50
Triscuit +	1	16	20
Uneeda +	1	20	30
Water Wafer +	1	8	30
Whole Wheat +	1	16	35
Zweibach +	1 slice	20	30

Eggs

ITEM	PORTION	CARBO-CALS	CALORIES
Boiled in Shell ○	1 medium	trace	77
Creamed eggs □	2 eggs, 2 tbs. sauce	52	270

ITEM	PORTION	CARBO-CALS	CALORIES
Deviled ☐	2 halves of med. egg	16	135
Dried, Whites ○	8 oz. cup	trace	223
Dried, Whole ○	8 oz. cup	trace	640
Dried, Yolks ○	8 oz. cup	trace	666
Duck Eggs ○	1 large	8	190
Fried ○	1 medium	2	100
Eggs A La Goldenrod +	6 tbs.	72	170
Omelette ○	1 med.	trace	106
Cheese (1 slice) ○	2 eggs	4	250
Spanish w/milk ☐	2 eggs	30	200
Poached ○	1 medium	trace	77
Poached in Jelly ☐	1 medium	30	100
Raw, Whole ○	1 medium	trace	77
Scrambled ○	1 medium	2	106
Stuffed ○	2 medium halves	8	125
Timbale ☐	5 tbs.	12	117
Turkey Eggs ○	1	10	248
White Only ○	1 medium egg	trace	15
Yolk Only ○	1 medium egg	trace	61

Fats

ITEM	PORTION	CARBO-CALS	CALORIES
Bacon Fat ○	1 tbs.	0	100
Beef Drippings ○	1 tbs.	0	50
Butter, salted ○	1 tbs.	0	100
salted patty ○	1 patty	0	50
sweet ○	1 tbs.	0	100
sweet, patty ○	1 patty	0	50
Chicken Fat ○	1 tbs.	0	100
Cod Liver Oil ○	1 tbs.	0	100
Corn Oil ○	1 tbs.	0	100
Cotton Seed Oil ○	1 tbs.	0	100
Crisco ○	8 oz. cup	0	1768
Crisco ○	1 tbs.	0	110
Cooking Fat ○	8 oz. cup	0	1768
Cooking Fat ○	1 tbs.	0	110
Ghee, High Moisture ○	3½ oz.	0	804
Low Moisture ○	3½ oz.	0	870
Halibut Oil ○	1 tbs.	0	100
Lard ○	8 oz. cup	0	1984

ITEM	PORTION	CARBO-CALS	CALORIES
Lard ○	1 tbs.	0	126
Margarine ○	1 tbs.	trace	100
Mineral Oil ○	1 tbs.	none	none
Oil, Cooking & Salad ○	8 oz. cup	0	1945
Oil, Cooking & Salad ○	1 tbs.	0	124
Oleomargarine ○	1 tbs.	0	101
Olive Oil ○	1 tbs.	0	125
Peanut Butter □	1 tbs.	12	93
Peanut Oil ○	1 tbs.	0	118
Vegetable ○	8 oz.	0	1768
Vegetable ○	1 tbs.	0	110
Viosterol	1 tbs.	0	0

Flours

ITEM	PORTION	CARBO-CALS	CALORIES
Barley +	8 oz. cup	360	420
Buckwheat, Dark-Sifted +	8 oz. cup	280	340
Buckwheat, Light-Sifted +	8 oz. cup	280	342
Cake Flour +	1 cup	290	350
Corn Flour, Dry Sifted +	8 oz. cup	450	470
Cornmeal, Degermed & Cooked +	8 oz. cup	100	120
Corn Soya +	8 oz. cup	70	125
Corn Soya Grits +	8 oz. cup	90	177
Corn Starch +	1 tbs.	28	37
Cracked Wheat +	8 oz. cup	400	468
Cracker Meal +	1 tbs.	28	60
Macaroni, cooked +	8 oz. cup	140	209
Noodles, cooked +	8 oz. cup	126	135
Noodles, fried +	1 oz.	64	88
Pancakes +			
Buckwheat +	4" diameter	24	47
	1 oz. cup	400	432
French +	4" diameter	30	62
Wheat +	4" diameter	28	50
Roman Meal +	8 oz. cup	260	350

ITEM	PORTION	CARBO-CALS	CALORIES
Rye, Light +	8 oz. cup	240	285
Soy Bean +	8 oz. cup	144	232
Starch, Pure +	8 oz. cup	460	464
Starch, Pure +	1 tbs.	28	29
Tortillas □	5" diameter	18	50
Wheat, all purpose +	8 oz. cup	320	401
Wheat Germ +	8 oz. cup	320	423

Fish

ITEM	PORTION	CARBO-CALS	CALORIES
Abalone			
Broiled ○	3½ oz.	trace	107
Canned ○	3½ oz.	trace	80
Dry ○	3½ oz.	trace	309
Raw ○	3½ oz.	trace	107
Anchovies ○	8 small fillets	trace	54
Paste ○	1 tsp.	trace	20
Bass ○			
Baked or Broiled ○	4 oz. portion	trace	180
Canned ○	4 oz. portion	trace	185
Raw ○	4 oz. portion	0	175
Bluefish ○			
Baked or Broiled ○	1 med. pc.	0	193
Baked or Broiled ○	1 pound	0	703
Fried ○	1 med. pc.	0	307
	1 pound	0	703
Butterfish ○			
Baked or Broiled ○	3 oz. portion	0	176
Catfish ○	3 oz. portion	0	168
Caviar ○	2 tbs.	4	70
Clams ○			
Canned ○	3 oz. solid & liquid	trace	44
Canned			
Cherrystone ○	4 oz. meat	16	90
Little Neck ○	4 oz. meat	16	90
Steamers ○	4 oz. meat	16	85
Raw, Meat Only ○	5 - 10	12	80
Steamed ○	6 w/butter	16	140
Stuffed, Baked □	2	40	180

ITEM	PORTION	CARBO-CALS	CALORIES
Cod ○	3½ oz. portion	0	98
Codfish ○			
Balls □	2 small balls	40	75
Baked +	1 medium	60	125
Creamed +	8 oz. cup	64	160
Dry □	1 oz. portion	20	106
Raw ○	4 oz. portion	trace	84
Salted ○	3½ oz. portion	trace	130
Steak ○	1 medium pc.	0	100
Crab			
Cracked ○	1 medium size	10	95
Hard Shell ○	3½ oz. portion	10	90
Soft Shell □	3½ oz. portion	32	90
Crabmeat, Cooked ○			
Canned ○	8 oz. meat	10	215
Deviled □	1 medium crab	40	200
Fresh ○	3 oz. meat	3	90
Salad □	4 oz. portion	30	150
Crab Jambalaya +	1 serving	60	180
Crab Paste ○	1 tsp.	trace	30
Croaker, Fresh ○	4 oz. portion	trace	109
Croquettes, Fish +	1 medium	64	120
Eel, Fresh ○	4 oz. portion	0	183
Eel, smoked ○	4 oz. portion	0	185
Finnan Haddie ○	4 oz. portion	0	100
Smoked ○	4 oz. portion	0	100
Fish			
Creamed □	½ cup	32	100
Cakes +	1	40	80
Sticks, Frozen +	4 oz.	30	90
Flounder ○	4 oz. portion	0	78
Frogs Legs ○	4 oz. portion	0	75
fried ○	4 oz. portion	4	170
Gefuelte Fish □	4 oz. portion	40	75
Haddock ○			
Cooked ○	1 fillet	0	158
Cooked ○	1 lb.	0	676
Creamed □	4 oz. portion	24	150
Fried □	1 fillet	32	165
Fried ○	1 lb.	trace	748

ITEM	PORTION	CARBO-CALS	CALORIES
Smoked ○	4 oz. portion	0	132
Halibut ○			
Broiled or cooked ○	1 steak (med.)	0	228
Broiled or cooked ○	1 lb. net	trace	827
Creamed ☐	4 oz. portion	24	170
Smoked ○	4 oz. portion	0	150
Herring ○			
Atlantic ○	4 oz. portion	0	216
Kippered ○	4 oz. portion	0	240
Lake ○	4 oz. portion	0	160
Pacific ○	4 oz. portion	0	105
Pickled ○	4 oz. portion	0	102
Pickled with sour cream ○	4 oz. portion	8	245
Smoked ○	4 oz. portion	0	240
Lobster ○			
Canned ○	3 oz. portion	trace	80
Canned ○	½ cup	trace	100
Creamed ☐	½ cup, 4 oz.	24	150
Fresh, Meat Only ○	3 oz.	trace	75
Fresh, w/2 tbs. butter ○	1	3	300
Baked or Broiled ○	1 average	3	120
Broiled ○	1 African Tail	0	150
Lobster Cantonese +	1 serving	30	200
Lobster Cocktail ☐	1 average	20	80
	½ cup meat, 2 tbs. sauce	32	90
	½ cup meat, wedge lemon	2	70
	½ cup meat, mayonnaise	trace	90
Lobster Newburgh ☐	½ cup	30	120
Lobster Paste ○	1 tsp.	trace	25
Lobster Thermador ☐	1 lobster	56	200
Lox, Nova Scotia, Smoked ○	3 oz. portion	0	285
Mackerel ○			
Canned, Atlantic ○	3 oz. portion	0	155
Canned, Pacific ○	3 oz. portion	0	153

ITEM	PORTION	CARBO-CALS	CALORIES
Fresh ○	3½ oz. portion	0	159
Salt ○	4 oz. portion	0	175
Mussels ○	6 medium size	trace	75
	1 lb.	28	250
Meskalunge ○	4 oz. portion	trace	100
Oysters			
Fried ☐	3 lg. pcs.	40	250
Raw, Blue Point ○	4 oz. meat	8	100
Raw, Blue Point ○	6-9 medium size	8	100
Oysters			
Raw, Cape Cod ○	4 oz. meat	8	100
Raw, Cape Cod ○	5-8 medium size	8	100
Stewed, Creamed ☐	8 oz. cup	40	250
Raw ☐	1 cup (13-19)	32	170
Scalloped +	6	120	250
Oyster Stew			
½ cream,			
½ milk ☐	8 oz. cup	88	200
Perch			
Lake ○	4 oz. portion	0	75
Sea ○	4 oz. portion	0	85
Fried ○	3 oz.	trace	85
Pickerel ○			
Sauteed ☐	4 oz.	24	208
Pike ○			
Northern ○	4 oz. portion	0	85
Wall Eyed ○	4 oz. portion	0	87
Porgy ○	4 oz. portion	0	110
Red Fish ○	4 oz. portion	0	100
Red Snapper ○	4 oz. portion	0	95
Cock Cod ○			
Broiled ○	4 oz.	0	122
Sauteed ○	4 oz.	0	173
Salmon ○			
Baked, Broiled ○	medium portion	0	204
Chinook ○	3 oz. portion	0	173
Chum ○	3 oz. portion	0	140
Cohoe ○	3 oz. portion	0	140
Creamed ☐	½ cup-4 oz.	64	200
Humpback ○	3 oz. portion	0	122
King ○	3 oz. portion	0	173

ITEM	PORTION	CARBO-CALS	CALORIES
Loaf □	1 average piece	20	200
Pink ○	3 oz. portion	0	122
Red ○	3 oz. portion	0	147
Silver ○	3 oz. portion	0	140
Smoked ○	3 oz. portion	0	285
Sand Dabs ○	2 medium pcs.	0	75
Sardines			
w/oil-drained solids ○	3 oz. portion	0	180
w/oil and solids ○	3 oz. portion	0	288
Natural Pack ○	3 oz. portion	0	171
Tomato Sauce Pack ○	3 oz. portion	4	184
Scallops			
Broiled □	4 oz. portion	10	175
Fried +	2-3 large pieces	56	295
Seafood au Gratin +	½ cup	48	300
Shad ○	4 oz. portion	0	191
Shad Roe ○	2 oz. portion	0	100
Shark's Fin, dried ○	3½ oz. portion	0	110
Shrimps			
Canned-Drained ○	3 oz. portion	trace	110
Canned-solids & liquids ○	3 oz. portion	0	76
Fresh ○	6 medium	trace	75
Fried □	6 medium-3½ oz.	32	100
Shrimp Scampi	6 in garlic butter	trace	175
Shrimp Cocktail □	1/3 cup w/sauce	40	80
Shrimp Creole +	6 shrimp w/sauce	100	160
Smelts ○	2 small size	0	50
Fried w/butter +	2-3	40	150
Snails ○	6 medium size	trace	52
Sole ○			
Fillet of ○	4 oz. portion	0	100
Sauteed ○	4 oz. portion	4	236
Squid, Raw ○	3½ oz. portion	0	78
Dried ○	3½ oz. portion	0	305
Sturgeon, Smoked ○	2½ oz. portion	0	100
Sword Fish ○	1 pc.	0	223
Trout ○			
Brook ○	3½ oz. portion	0	50

ITEM	PORTION	CARBO-CALS	CALORIES
Brook, smoked ○	3 oz. portion	0	100
Lake ○	3 oz. portion	0	60
Lake, smoked ○	3 oz. portion	0	110
Tuna ○			
Canned, Drained ○	3 oz. portion	0	170
Canned, w/oil			
(Wet Pack) ○	3 oz. portion	0	247
Creamed ○	½ cup - 4 oz.	8	270
Fresh ○	3 oz. portion	0	150
Smoked ○	2½ oz. portion	0	125
Tuna Casserole			
w/noodles +	1 average portion	100	300
Turtle ○	½ cup - 4 oz.	0	160
Whale Meat ○	3½ oz. portion	0	116
Whitefish ○			
Broiled ○	4 oz. portion	0	125
Fried ○	4 oz. portion	0	200
Baked, Stuffed □	1 serving	44	260

Fruits

ITEM	PORTION	CARBO-CALS	CALORIES
Apple +	1 large	100	160
Apple +	1 medium	64	85
Apple +	1 small	44	60
Baked w/sugar +	1 medium	150	200
Baked w/sugar +	1 large	200	260
Dried, Cooked,			
unsweetened +	¼ cup	92	102
Dried, Cooked,			
sweetened +	¼ cup	100	160
Applesauce +			
Canned, Infant +	1 oz. strained	20	25
Sweetened +	8 oz. cup	200	260
Unsweetened +	8 oz. cup	104	120
Apricots □			
Canned, Infant □	1 oz. strained	40	17
Canned, Syrup			
Pack +	4 med. size halves	80	97
Canned, Syrup			
Pack +	8 oz. cup halves	200	205

ITEM	PORTION	CARBO-CALS	CALORIES
Canned, Water Pack ☐	8 oz. cup halves	80	77
Dried +	8 oz. cup halves	360	423
Dried, Cooked +	½ cup sweetened	200	220
Dried, Cooked +	½ cup unsweetened	120	130
Fresh ☐	3 medium size	40	54
Stewed +	8 oz. cup	360	400
Avocado, California ☐	½ pear	24	279
Avocado, California ☐	8 oz. cup of cubes	36	372
Avocado, Florida +	½ pear	44	279
Avocado, Florida +	8 oz. cup of cubes	52	372
Bananas +	1 large	115	120
Bananas +	1 medium	100	110
Diced +	1 cup	125	136
Fried +	1 medium	130	140
Sliced +	1 cup	140	150
Fritter +		44	80
Blackberries ☐	1 cup	72	82
Canned,			
Syrup Pack +	8 oz. cup	180	216
Water Pack ☐	8 oz. cup	88	104
Low Calorie,			
Canned ☐	1 cup	72	80
Blueberries ☐	1 cup	80	85
Canned,			
Syrup Pack +	8 oz. cup	240	245
Water Pack ☐	8 oz. cup	80	90
Frozen,			
unsweetened ☐	3 oz.	40	52
Frozen,			
sweetened +	1 cup	150	160
Canned,			
Low Calorie ☐	1 cup	68	80
Boysenberries ☐			
Frozen,			
sweetened +	1 cup	140	160
Frozen,			
unsweetened ☐	1 cup	44	70
Cantaloupe ☐	½ of medium size	32	37
	1 cup diced	22	30
Casaba Melon ☐	1 wedge	40	52

ITEM	PORTION	CARBO-CALS	CALORIES
Cherries +			
Canned +	8 oz. cup	110	122
Fresh, pitted +	1 cup	80	94
Fresh +	1 cup	60	65
Maraschino +	1 medium size	20	25
Canned, Bing,			
Low Calorie +	1 cup	88	100
Canned, Bing,			
in syrup +	1 cup	240	300
Canned, Red Sour +	1 cup	96	120
Canned,			
Royale Anne +	1 cup	190	210
Canned, Royale Anne,			
Low Calorie +	1 cup	84	90
Citron, Dried +	1 pc.	45	50
Cocoanut ☐	1 medium piece	24	161
Shredded ☐	8 oz. cup	52	349
Dried, Shredded,			
Sweetened +	1 cup	120	900
Crab Apple ☐	1 medium size	12	30
Cranberries ☐	8 oz. cup	44	54
Cranberry Relish			
w/orange +	¼ cup	100	120
Currants +	8 oz. cup	48	60
Cooked, sweetened +	8 oz. cup	90	125
Dried +	2 tbs.	80	85
Cranberry Sauce,			
sweetened +	8 oz. cup	400	549
Dates +	3 or 4	90	100
Figs +	2 or 3 small size	80	90
Canned, w/syrup +	3 figs/2 tbs. syrup	120	129
Canned, w/syrup +	8 oz. cup	290	300
Dried +	1 large size	44	57
Canned,			
Low Calorie ☐	½ cup	40	50
Fruit Cocktail ☐	¾ cup-6 oz.	100	110
Canned,			
Low Calorie ☐	1 cup	40	50
Canned +	3 tbs.	120	130
Fruits for Salad ☐			
Canned +	3 tbs.	110	125

ITEM	PORTION	CARBO-CALS	CALORIES
Canned,			
Low Calorie ☐	⅔ cup	28	35
Gooseberries ☐	8 oz. cup	50	59
Grandilla (Passion			
Fruit) ☐	3½ oz. pulp & seeds	85	100
Grapes +			
Concord +	4 oz.	60	80
Delaware +	4 oz.	60	80
Flame Tokay +	8 oz. cup	128	150
Malaga +	8 oz. cup	128	150
Muscat +	8 oz. cup	128	150
Niagara +	1 bunch	60	80
Sultana +	8 oz. cup	128	150
Thompson Seedless +	8 oz. cup	120	140
Tokay +	8 oz. cup	128	150
Canned,			
with syrup +	1 cup	180	200
Canned,			
with water +	1 cup	88	100
Grapefruit ☐	½ large	88	104
Grapefruit ☐	½ medium	72	75
Grapefruit ☐	½ small	45	49
Canned,			
sweetened +	8 oz. cup	160	181
Canned,			
unsweetened ☐	8 oz. cup	80	90
Sections ☐	8 oz. cup	70	77
Fresh Pink ☐	½ medium	65	75
Guavas ☐	1 medium	40	49
Honeydew Melon ☐	1 medium wedge	45	49
Huckleberries ☐	8 oz. cup	80	85
Kumquat ☐	3½ oz. piece	68	75
Kumquat ☐	1 tbs.	20	25
Kumquat ☐	5-6	40	45
Lemon ☐	1 medium	32	40
Lime ☐	1-2	24	26
Loganberries ☐	⅔ cup	60	70
Canned +	8 oz. cup	100	104
Dried +	3½ oz. portion	270	286
Loquat ☐	6-8	40	48
Lotus Seeds +	3½ oz. portion	300	350

ITEM	PORTION	CARBO-CALS	CALORIES
Mamey Apple ☐	3½ oz. portion	45	51
Mangoes ☐	1 medium	44	48
Muskmelon ☐	½ of medium	32	37
Nectarine ☐	1 medium	32	38
Orange ☐	Large	90	106
Orange ☐	medium	65	70
Orange ☐	small	44	49
Sections ☐	8 oz. cup	80	87
Orange & Grapefruit sections ☐	8 oz. cup	70	82
Papaya, Fresh ☐	8 oz. cup of cubes	65	71
Passion Fruit +	3½ oz. pulp & seeds	85	100
Peach ☐	1 medium size	40	46
Sliced ☐	8 oz. cup	72	77
Canned, Infant ☐	1 oz. strained	20	25
Canned, Syrup Pack +	8 oz. cup	150	174
Canned, Syrup Pack +	2 medium halves w/syrup	70	79
Canned, Water Pack ☐	8 oz. cup	60	66
Dried, Sulphured, no sugar +	8 oz. cup	240	320
Dried, Sulphured, w/sugar +	8 oz. cup	350	366
Dried +	1 cup	400	450
Pears +	1 medium	90	95
Fresh, quarters +	8 oz. medium	110	120
Canned, Infant ☐	1 oz. strained	12	15
Canned, Syrup Pack +	8 oz. cup	170	180
Canned, Syrup Pack +	2 med. halves	70	79
Canned, Water Packed ☐	8 oz. cup	70	75
Spiced, w/syrup +	1 med. size	70	79
Canned, Low Calorie ☐	1 cup	56	60
Persian Melon ☐	1 medium wedge	48	52
Persimmons +	8 oz. medium	240	250

ITEM	PORTION	CARBO-CALS	CALORIES
Pineapple ☐			
Canned,			
Syrup Pack +	2 small slices	90	95
Canned,			
Syrup Pack +	1 large slice	90	95
Fresh, Diced ☐	8 oz. cup	70	74
Fresh, Sliced ☐	1 slice medium	40	44
Frozen +	4 oz. package	112	118
Canned,			
Low Calorie ☐	½ cup	44	50
Candied +	1 slice	120	150
Pitanga ☐	3½ oz.	40	51
Plantain +	3½ oz.	110	119
Plums ☐	1 medium	25	29
Fresh, Halves ☐	8 oz. cup	85	94
Canned,	8 oz. cup	200	210
Low Calorie ☐	1 cup	40	50
Poka, Hawaiian ☐	1 cup	44	60
Pomegranate +	1 medium size	70	75
Prickly Pear ☐	1 medium size	20	52
Prunes +			
Canned, Infant +	1 oz. strained	28	28
Cooked, no sugar +	8 oz. cup	160	200
Cooked, w/sugar +	8 oz. cup	300	320
Dried, small +	1	12	14
Dried +	8 oz. cup	350	375
Pummelo ☐	3½ oz. portion	40	48
Quince ☐	1 medium size	40	45
Raisins +	4	12	14
Sugar Added +	8 oz. cup	520	572
Dried +	8 oz. cup	400	429
Dried +	1 tbs.	20	26
Raspberries ☐			
Canned +	8 oz. cup	220	250
Fresh, Black ☐	8 oz. cup	84	100
Fresh, Red ☐	8 oz. cup	65	70
Frozen +	3 oz. package	95	126
Canned,			
With Water ☐	24	35	
Rhubarb ☐	8 oz. cup	16	19
Roseapple ☐	3½ oz. portion	50	56

ITEM	PORTION	CARBO-CALS	CALORIES
Sapodilla ☐	3½ oz. portion	80	89
Sapote +	3½ oz. portion	110	125
Soursop ☐	3½ oz. portion	60	65
Strawberries ☐	8 oz. cup	52	54
Frozen +	3 oz. package	80	90
Fresh ☐	5 large	20	25
Tangerine ☐	1 medium size	30	35
Watermelon ☐	½ slice	40	45
	wedge, medium	85	100
Balls or Cubes ☐	½ cup	28	35

Ice Cream

ITEM	PORTION	CARBO-CALS	CALORIES
Banana Ice Cream +	1 scoop - ½ cup	72	292
Banana Split (Royal) +	Fountain size	400	1165
Black & White Soda +	Fountain size	120	308
Butter Almond +	1 scoop - ½ cup	80	297
Butter Pecan +	1 scoop - ½ cup	80	297
Butterscotch Ice Cream +	1 scoop - ½ cup	70	294
Butterscotch Ice Cream Sundae +	Fountain size	150	250
Caramel Ice Cream +	1 scoop - ½ cup	70	296
Cherry Ice +	1 scoop - ½ cup	110	118
Cherry Ice Cream +	1 scoop - ½ cup	70	295
Cherry Soda +	Fountain size	115	306
Cherry-Vanilla Ice Cream +	1 scoop - ½ cup	70	294
Chocolate Chip Ice Cream +	1 scoop - ½ cup	90	298
Chocolate Covered Pop, Ice Cream +	1 regular pop	90	324
Chocolate Ice Cream +	1 scoop - ½ cup	80	298
Chocolate Ice Cream Soda +	Fountain size	160	320
Chocolate Malted Milk	Fountain size	140	305
w/ice cream +		220	600
Chocolate Pop +	1 regular pop	80	318
Chocolate Sundae +			
Fancy-			

ITEM	PORTION	CARBO-CALS	CALORIES
Fountain Size +		150	330
Plain +	Fountain size	130	280
Vanilla			
Ice Cream +	Fountain size	200	420
Chocolate			
Ice Cream +	Fountain size	220	440
Cocoanut Covered			
Pop +	1 regular pop	160	315
Coffee Ice Cream +	1 scoop - ½ cup	78	292
Coffee Soda +	Fountain size	115	308
Cone, Ice Cream +	1 average	12	45
(NOTE: - Refer to Ice Cream flavor and add for cone)			
Custard, frozen +	1 scoop - ½ cup	70	150
Dixie cup +	1 regular dixie	65	206
All Ice Cream			
Dixie +	1 regular dixie	75	276
Sundae +	1 regular dixie	80	294
Fudge Pop,			
Ice Cream +	1 regular pop	90	318
Fudge Sundae +			
Fancy +	Fountain size	120	330
Plain +	Fountain size	108	280
Hot Fancy +	Fountain size	125	340
Hot Plain +	Fountain size	110	285
Lemon Ice +	1 scoop - ½ cup	110	116
Lemon Ice Cream +	1 scoop - ½ cup	70	292
Malted Milks +	Fountain size	140	305
Chocolate Shake +	Fountain size	200	305
Chocolate Ice Cream			
Shake +	Fountain size	280	600
Misc. Flavors &			
Ice Cream +	Fountain size	260	595
Malted Milk			
Powder +	1 tbsp.	28	50
Maple Mousse +	Fountain size	200	356
Maple Walnut			
Sundae +			
Fancy +	Fountain size	118	325
Plain +	Fountain size	90	275
Marshmallow Sundae +			
Fancy +	Fountain size	110	329

ITEM	PORTION	CARBO-CALS	CALORIES
Fancy with nuts +	Fountain size	120	337
Plain +	Fountain size	90	278
Plain with nuts +	Fountain size	95	283
Nesselrode			
Ice Cream +	1 scoop - ½ cup	80	297
Orange Ice +	1 scoop - ½ cup	110	117
Parfait +			
Coffee +	1 regular	60	200
Maple +	1 regular	80	240
Peach Ice Cream +	1 scoop - ½ cup	70	295
Peace Ice Cream			
Soda +	Fountain size	75	311
Pie on Stick			
Ice Cream +	1 regular pie	90	324
Pineapple			
Ice Cream +	½ cup - 4 oz.	70	250
Pineapple Ice Cream			
Soda +	Fountain size	90	314
Pineapple Sundae +			
Fancy +	Fountain size	160	327
Plain +	Fountain size	150	276
Ice Pop +	1 regular pop	100	118
Raspberry Ice +	1 scoop - ½ cup	110	120
Sandwich, Ice Cream +	1 regular sandwich	110	255
Sherbet +			
with milk +	¼ pint	100	135
with water +	¼ pint	75	90
Ice Cream Sodas +			
Artificial flavors +	1 fountain serving	150	300
Chocolate flavor +	1 fountain serving	150	320
Fresh Fruit Flavor +	1 fountain serving	150	310
with Chocolate			
Ice Cream +	1 fountain serving	160	320
Tutti Frutti			
Ice Cream +	1 scoop - ½ cup	60	150
Vanilla +	1 scoop - ½ cup	80	214
Vanilla Fudge			
Ice Cream +	1 scoop - ½ cup	90	220
Vanilla Fudge Pop +	1 regular pop	90	220
Vanilla Malted,			

ITEM	PORTION	CARBO-CALS	CALORIES
Plain +	Fountain size	110	250
with ice cream +	Fountain size	200	440
Walnut Sundae,			
Plain +	Fountain size	120	274
Fancy +	Fountain size	150	325

Jams and Jellies

ITEM	PORTION	CARBO-CALS	CALORIES
Apple Butter +	1 tbs.	28	35
Blackberry Jam +	1 tbs.	56	60
Blackberry Jelly +	1 tbs.	52	60
Coffee Jelly +	1 tbs.	40	48
Cranberry Jelly +	1 tbs.	32	35
Currant Jelly +	1 tbs.	52	60
Fruit Jellies (Most) +	1 tbs.	40	50
Guava Butter +	1 tbs.	40	50
Guava Jelly +	1 tbs.	52	60
Grape Jelly +	1 tbs.	52	60
Jams, (Most) +	1 tbs.	52	55
Lemon Jelly +	1 tbs.	52	60
Marmalade +	1 tbs.	56	60
Marmalade, Papaya +	1 tbs.	58	60
Plum Jam +	1 tbs.	52	55
Preserves (Most) +	1 tbs.	52	55
Strawberry Jam +	1 tbs.	52	55

Meats

ITEM	PORTION	CARBO-CALS	CALORIES
BEEF ○			
Canned, Infant ○	1 oz. strained	0	30
Canned, Roast Beef ○	3 oz. portion	0	189
Brains ○	⅔ cup	6	400
Brisket ○	3½ oz.	0	380
Chipped Beef ○	8 oz. cup	0	336
with cream □	½ cup	24	175
Chuck or Cooked			
Beef ○	3½ oz. without bone	0	421
Corned Beef ○			
Boiled ○	1 med. pc.	0	100

ITEM	PORTION	CARBO-CALS	CALORIES
Canned, Lean ◯	3 oz.	0	159
Canned, Medium Fat ◯	3 oz.	0	182
Canned, Fat ◯	3 oz.	0	221
Corned and Hash ☐	1 cup	80	320
Croquettes, Beef ☐	1 medium	36	280
Filet Mignon ◯	3½ oz. portion	0	224
Flank and Cooked Beef ◯	3½ oz. without bone	0	235
Hamburger ◯	1 lb. portion	0	1654
Hamburger ◯	3 oz. portion	0	316
Dried Beef ◯	1 cup	0	336
Dried Beef ◯	2 oz. portion	0	115
Heart, Beef ◯	3 oz. portion	2	90
Lean ◯	3 oz. portion	2	164
Braised ◯	3 oz. portion	3	170
Kidney Beef ◯	½ cup portion	4	160
Liver, cooked ☐	3½ oz.	24	207
Infant ◯	1 oz. strained	7	30
Lung, Beef ◯	4 oz. portion	4	105
Meat Balls ◯	3 oz.	0	316
Meat Loaf ☐	1 slice, 3 oz.	44	320
Porterhouse Steak, Cooked ◯			
with bone ◯	1 lb.	0	895
without bone ◯	1 lb.	0	1100
without bone ◯	3½ oz.	0	242
Pot Pie +	4¼" diameter	148	450
Pot Roast, Cooked ◯	3½ oz. portion	0	298
Rib Roast, Cooked ◯			
with bone ◯	1 lb.	0	1050
without bone ◯	1 lb.	0	1189
without bone ◯	3½ oz.	0	262
Round Steak, Regular, Cooked ◯			
without bone ◯	1 lb.	0	1040
without bone ◯	3½ oz.	0	229
Round Steak, Bottom, Cooked ◯			
with bone ◯	1 lb.	0	917

ITEM	PORTION	CARBO-CALS	CALORIES
without bone ○	1 lb.	0	1281
without bone ○	3½ oz.	0	250
Rump, Cooked ○			
with bone ○	1 lb.	0	850
without bone ○	1 lb.	0	1067
without bone ○	3½ oz.	0	235
Sirloin, Cooked ○			
with bone ○	1 lb.	0	800
without bone ○	1 lb.	0	944
without bone ○	3½ oz.	0	200
Stew, Beef ○	1 cup	0	350
Stew, Beef and			
Vegetable +	8 oz. cup	80	252
Sweetbreads, broiled ○	½ cup	0	100
creamed □	½ cup	24	300
Swiss Steak +	3½ oz.	68	300
T Bone Steak ○	3½ oz. portion	0	247
Tenderloin Steak ○	3½ oz. portion	0	224
Tongue, Beef,			
Medium Fat ○	3 oz.	trace	174
Pickled ○	1 tbs.	trace	32
Canned ○	4 oz. portion	trace	252
Tripe ○	½ cup	0	100
Pickled ○	3½ oz.	trace	88
LAMB			
Canned, Infant ○	1 oz. strained	0	30
Curry, Lamb +	½ cup	88	400
Kidneys ○	½ cup	4	118
Chops ○			
Broiled, without			
bone ○	3½ oz.	0	223
Fried, without bone ○	3½ oz.	0	270
Rib Chops, Broiled ○	3½ oz.	0	291
Roast Leg ○			
with bone ○	1 lb.	0	720
without bone ○	1 lb.	0	885
without bone ○	3½ oz.	0	195
Shish Kebab, Lamb ○	3½ oz.	0	300
Shoulder Roast ○			
without bone ○	1 lb.	0	1551

ITEM	PORTION	CARBO-CALS	CALORIES
without bone ○	3 oz.	0	293
with bone ○	1 lb.	0	1160
Sirloin Chops ○	1 medium chop	0	110
Stew, Lamb ○	8 oz. cup	0	300
Stew, Lamb with vegetables +	8 oz. cup	44	450
Chops or Roast Mutton			
thin fat ○	3½ oz.	0	206
medium fat ○	3½ oz.	0	317
LIVERS			
Canned, Infant ○	3½ oz.	6	100
Canned, Infant ○	1 oz.	trace	30
Beef Liver ☐	3½ oz.	24	160
Calves Liver ☐	3½ oz. portion	16	140
Chicken Liver			
Broiled ○	3½ oz.	6	141
Raw ○	3½ oz.	6	120
Sauteed ☐	3½ oz.	12	155
Chicken Liver, Chopped ☐	3 oz. portion	12	150
Goose Liver ☐	2 medium	12	150
Lamb or Sheep ☐	3 oz. portion	16	116
	1 slice	12	90
Liverwurst ○	2 oz. slice	2	150
Pork ○	1 slice	8	320
Spread, Liver ○	2 tbs./1 oz.	trace	95
Steer ☐	3 oz. portion	16	119
PORK, HAM			
Baked ○	1 medium slice	0	265
Boiled, with bone ◉	1 lb.	0	1432
Boiled, without bone ○	1 lb.	0	1818
Boiled, without bone ○	3 oz.	0	338
Boiled, Luncheon ○	2 oz.	0	172
Deviled ○	1 tbs.	4	50
Fried ○	3 oz. portion	0	342
Hocks ○	3 oz. portion	0	340
Loaf ○	3 oz. portion	0	355
Luncheon, Canned & Spiced ○	3 oz.	trace	246

ITEM	PORTION	CARBO- CALS	CALORIES
Picnic, Shoulder,			
Fresh ○	3½ oz.	trace	246
Prosciutto ○	1½ oz.	0	170
Smoked, with bone ○	1 lb.	trace	1496
Smoked,			
without bone ○	1 lb.	trace	1804
Smoked,			
without bone ○	3 oz.	trace	339
Spiced, Fresh,			
Canned ○	2 oz.	trace	165
Heart, Pork ○	3 oz. portion	trace	150
Kidneys, Pork ○	½ cup	trace	129
Pigs Feet ○			
Boiled ○	4 oz.	0	185
Pickled ○	4 oz. portion	trace	230
Boston Butt ○	3½ oz. portion	trace	283
Canned,			
Infant Pork ○	1 oz. strained	0	36
Canned, Spiced ○	2 oz. portion	0	165
Chops ○			
with bone ○	1 lb.	0	1149
Loin, Center Cut,			
without bone ○	1 lb.	0	1135
Loin, Center Cut,			
with bone ○	3 oz. portion	0	210
without bone ○	3½ oz. portion	0	250
Carcass			
Medium Fat ○	3½ oz. portion	0	457
Thin ○	3½ oz. portion	0	376
Leg Roast ○	3 oz. portion	0	270
Loin ○			
Roasted with			
bone ○	1 lb.	0	1149
Roasted without			
bone ○	1 lb.	0	1508
Roasted, 1 chop ○	3½ oz.	0	293
Roasted, without	3 oz. portion	0	284
bone ○			
Pork ○			
Salt Pork ○	3 oz. portion	0	200
Sirloin Pork ○	3½ oz. portion	0	227

ITEM		PORTION	CARBO-CALS	CALORIES
Spareribs	○	3½ oz. medium	0	351
Tenderloin, Pork	○	3½ oz. portion	0	239
Tongue	○	3½ oz. portion	trace	214
POULTRY AND				
GAME	○			
Chicken	○			
Boiled	○	4 oz. serving	0	75
Broiled	○	½ medium size	0	210
Canned, Boned	○	3 oz.	trace	169
Creamed	☐	½ cup - 4 oz.	20	216
Croquettes	+	1 medium size	30	105
Fat	○	1 tbs.	0	100
Fried	○	5 oz.	10	204
Fried	○	1 leg	5	65
Fried	☐	8 oz. ½ medium	25	255
Gizzard	○	3½ oz. serving	0	116
Heart	○	3 oz. pc.	4	134
Liver, Broiled	○	3½ oz. serving	trace	141
Raw	○	3 oz. serving	trace	120
Sauteed	○	3 oz. serving	trace	155
Raw, Broilers	○	½ bird boned	0	332
Raw, Friers,				
Boned	○	1 breast	0	210
Raw, Roasters,				
Boned	○	4 oz. pc.	0	227
Raw, Stewing Hen,				
Boned	○	4 oz. pc.	0	342
Chicken A La King	☐	½ cup	24	218
Chicken Paprikash	☐	Small serving	20	200
Chicken Pie	+	Small Pie	80	400
Chicken TV Dinner	+	1	160	500
Duck	○			
Gizzard	○	3½ oz. serving	0	127
Raw	○	3½ oz. serving	0	326
Raw, Dried and				
Salted	○	3½ oz. serving	0	413
Roasted, Boned	○	4 oz. piece	0	325
Goose	○			
Gizzard	○	3½ oz. serving	0	139
Raw	○	3½ oz. serving	0	354
Roasted, Boned	○	4 oz. piece	0	315

ITEM	PORTION	CARBO-CALS	CALORIES
Pate Maison □	3 oz. portion	20	200
Pate De Fois Gras ○	1 tbs.	3	75
Pheasant, Roasted, Boned ○	4 oz. piece	0	150
Quail, Broiled ○	4 oz. portion	0	150
Squab, Broiled boned ○	3½ oz. portion	0	279
Stuffing, Meat or Poultry +	½ cup	112	330
Turkey			
All Dark ○	4 oz. serving	0	327
All White ○	4 oz. serving	0	280
Gizzard ○	3½ oz. serving	0	188
Raw, Medium Fat ○	4 oz. piece	0	304
Roasted ○	4 oz. piece	0	318
Creamed on Toast +	1 cup	52	400
Pot Pie +	1 pie	160	420
VEAL			
Canned, Infant ○	1 oz. strained	0	24
Carcass ○			
Thin ○	3½ oz. portion	0	156
Medium Fat ○	3½ oz. portion	0	190
MISC.			
Frankfurter ○	1 average	4	124
Hash			
Canned, Corned Beef □	3 oz.	28	155
Horsemeat ○	3½ oz. portion	4	218
Pastrami ○	2 medium slices	0	170
Rabbit ○	3 oz. portion	0	162
Stew □	1 cup	44	560
Sausages			
Cervelat ○	1 medium piece	4	50
Pork Links ○	1 link	0	63
Salami □	8 oz.	12	467
Vienna Sausage ○	8 oz. portion	3	488
Polish ○	8 oz.	4	450
Pork Sausage ○	4 oz. portion	trace	540
Head Cheese, Sausage ○	3 oz. piece	0	70
Tongue, Canned ○	3 oz.	trace	210

ITEM	PORTION	CARBO-CALS	CALORIES
Venison ○	4 oz. slice	0	225
Wienerschnitzel ○	4 oz. slice	4	275

Milk

ITEM	PORTION	CARBO-CALS	CALORIES
Buttermilk +	8 oz. glass	48	90
Cultured +	8 oz. glass	48	85
Acidophilus Milk +	8 oz. cup	40	100
Chocolate Milk +			
all milk +	8 oz. glass	96	185
skimmed milk +	8 oz. glass	104	110
Cocoa			
Whole milk +	8 oz. glass	68	178
skimmed milk +	8 oz. glass	75	106
Cocoamalt, all milk +	1 cup	130	280
Cocoa Powder, Dry +	1 tbs.	12	32
Cocoanut milk +	8 oz. glass	48	60
Condensed Milk +	1 tbs.	40	62
Sweetened +	1 cup	680	981
Cream,			
Coffee or light □	½ pint	8	489
	1 tbs.	2	30
Half and Half □	1 cup	44	384
Heavy ○	1 tbs.	trace	50
Whipping ○	1 tbs.	trace	49
	½ pint	8	780
Whipped ○	1 pint volume	4	78
Whipped ○	1 tbs.	trace	25
Evaporated Milk +	1 tbs.	6	20
Evaporated Milk +	1 cup	96	345
half water +	1 cup	48	170
Goat's Milk +	8 oz. cup	44	165
Half and Half □	8 oz. cup	4	330
Non-Fat Milk			
Dry +	1 cup	160	250
Dry +	1 tbs.	10	18
Ovaltine, all milk +	8 oz.	84	240
skimmed milk +	8 oz.	95	175
Sheep's Milk □	½ cup	18	110

ITEM	PORTION	CARBO-CALS	CALORIES
Skimmed Milk +	8 oz. glass	50	85
Sour Cream ☐	1 tbs.	2	58
Sour Cream ☐	1 cup	32	900
Soy Bean Milk ☐	8 oz. cup	16	75
Whole Milk +			
Dry	1 tbs.	8	40
Regular	8 oz. glass	48	165
Yogurt +	1 cup	52	120

Nuts

ITEM	PORTION	CARBO-CALS	CALORIES
Almonds +			
Shelled +	½ cup	56	424
In Shell +	1 cup	32	238
Salted +	12-15	12	100
Brazil +			
Shelled +	½ cup	28	452
In Shell +	1 cup	24	394
Shelled +	6	12	210
Butter +	4 - 6	4	100
Cashew +	1 oz. roasted	32	164
Roasted +	1 cup	140	680
Roasted +	6 - 8	12	80
Chestnut +	5 - 6	52	63
Filbert +	10 - 12	8	100
Hazel +	10 - 12	8	110
Hickory +	12 - 15	8	100
Lichee Nuts +			
Fresh +	3½ oz.	40	64
Dried +	3½ oz.	200	277
Lotus Seeds +	3½ oz.	50	351
Macadamia Nuts +	¼ cup	20	245
Mixed Nuts +	6 - 8	8	100
Peanuts +			
Chopped +	1 tbs.	8	50
Shelled +	1 cup	90	805
In Shell +	12 - 15	12	100
Spanish +	2 tbs.	10	90

ITEM	PORTION	CARBO-CALS	CALORIES
Pecans +			
Halves +	1 cup	56	752
chopped +	1 tbs.	4	52
	12 nutmeats	8	112
Pine Nuts +	12 - 15	12	100
	½ cup salted	20	150
Pistachio +	12 medium nuts	4	100
	20 nuts	6	180
Sesame Seeds, Whole +	3½ oz.	80	568
Walnuts +			
Black +	11 meats	12	100
Black, Chopped +	1 tbs.	4	50
English +	10 - 12	10	106
	1½ tbs. chopped	10	106
Persian +	10 - 12	10	105
	1½ tbs. chopped	10	100

Pies

PORTIONS FOR ALL PIES: BETWEEN 1/7 and 1/8 SECTION

Apple +		200	331
Apricot +		230	328
Banana Cream +		160	340
Berry, Most Pies +		180	300
Blackberry +		180	296
Blueberry +		185	291
Butterscotch +		168	265
Cheese +		160	330
Cherry +		200	340
Chocolate Chiffon,			
Whipped Cream +		140	220
Chocolate Meringue +		150	240
Cocoanut Custard +		130	266
Cream +		170	260
Custard Cream +		130	265
Gooseberry +		120	298
Lemon Chiffon +		150	300
Lemon Meringue +		170	302
Mince +		230	341

ITEM	PORTION	CARBO-CALS	CALORIES
Peach +		230	330
Peach Cream +		240	355
Pecan +		235	350
Pineapple +		150	340
Pineapple Cheese +		165	340
Pineapple Cream +		200	350
Prune +		210	330
Pumpkin +		130	263
Raisin +		250	325
Rhubarb +		200	328
Shoofly +		200	300
Strawberry +		200	310
Strawberry Cream +		225	350
Pie Crust +			
Double Bottom +		572	720
Bottom Crust +		280	380
Graham Cracker (Bottom) +		260	345

Puddings

ITEM	PORTION	CARBO-CALS	CALORIES
Apple Betty +	8 oz. cup	280	344
Apple Dumpling +	1 med. size pc.	200	345
Apple Snow +	½ cup	70	75
Apricot Whip +	½ cup	85	100
Banana Custard +	½ cup	80	125
Banana Whip +	½ cup	60	85
Bavarian Orange +	1 serving	160	185
Blanc Mange +	½ cup	80	130
Chocolate +	½ cup	100	138
Vanilla +	½ cup	90	135
Bread +	½ cup	112	150
Brown Betty +	8 oz. cup	140	344
Butterscotch +	½ cup	120	175
Sugar Free ☐	½ cup	36	90
Caramel +	½ cup	112	170
Chocolate +	½ cup	120	175
Skim Milk +	½ cup	120	150
Corn Puddings, Southern +	½ cup	52	100

ITEM	PORTION	CARBO-CALS	CALORIES
Corn Starch,			
Most Flavors +	½ cup	110	170
Butterscotch +	½ cup	74	260
Chocolate +	½ cup	74	270
Vanilla +	½ cup	80	250
Cottage Pudding +	1 pc.	160	240
w/2 tbs. lemon			
sauce +	1 pc.	240	300
Custard □	½ cup	56	160
Canned, Instant □	1 oz. strained	10	31
Caramel □	½ cup	48	140
Egg □	½ cup	40	145
Frozen □	1 scoop	50	150
Date Torte,			
with Cream +	½ cup	250	400
Fig +	½ cup	200	300
Floating Island □	½ cup	50	150
Frozen Custard □	1 scoop	50	150
Gelatin,			
Ready-to-serve ○	8 oz. cup	0	155
with fruit +	8 oz. cup	110	172
Fruit Jello,			
All Flavors +	8 oz.	100	230
Indian, Baked □	½ cup	50	150
Junket □	½ cup	20	100
Lemon Spunge +	½ cup	104	125
with custard sauce	½ cup	160	220
Plum, No Sauce +	½ cup	100	150
Prune Whip +	½ cup	100	200
Rice +	½ cup	68	128
Custard +		100	152
with raisins +	½ cup	128	175
Tapioca +	½ cup	180	260
Vanilla +	½ cup	96	138

Salads

Apple Carrot □	½ cup	46	270
Asparagus Tips □	5 med. spears	14	35

ITEM	PORTION	CARBO-CALS	CALORIES
Avocado ☐	½ of med. pear	35	279
Cubed ☐	½ cup	20	186
with tomato &			
cottage cheese ☐		36	220
Banana +	1 medium used	100	310
Banana and nut +	½ banana used	60	200
Banana and Orange +	½ of each	88	210
Cabbage Slaw ☐	6 tbs.	20	50
Carrot-Raisin +	3 tbs.	112	150
Chicken Salad ☐	½ cup chicken	10	230
Crab Meat ☐	½ cup packed	12	100
Dandelion Greens ☐	1 cup packed	8	100
Deviled Meat ☐	2 tbs. rounded used	trace	150
Eggs			
Deviled ☐	2 halves used	10	148
Sliced ☐	1 medium used	trace	85
Egg and Tomato ☐	½ cup of each	16	180
Endive ☐	1 cup packed	30	50
and grapefruit ☐	1 cup packed	50	65
Escarole ☐	1 cup packed	25	50
Fig, Fresh +	3 small used	85	100
Fruit Combination			
Canned +	¾ cup	90	135
Fresh +	¾ cup	80	95
Canned +	3 tbs.	120	150
Canned,			
Low Calorie ☐	⅔ cup	28	50
Herring ☐	½ cup	20	115
Lettuce ☐	4 leaves used	trace	7
and tomato ☐	1 cup heaped	20	25
with French Dressing			
Wedge ☐		28	130
Lobster ☐	3 oz. portion used	20	85
Canned ☐	3 oz. portion	25	90
Macaroni +	1 cup	200	310
Orange and Grapefruit			
with dressing ☐	½ cup	40	200
Pineapple ☐	½ cup used	45	115
and Cheese ☐	¾ cup portion	70	218
Potato +	½ cup	52	100

ITEM	PORTION	CARBO-CALS	CALORIES
Prunes, Stuffed with Cottage Cheese +	4	112	
Salmon ☐	3 oz. used	10	200
Sardine ☐	3 oz. used	8	200
Seafood Combination ☐	½ cup packed	8	100
Shrimp ☐	½ cup packed	5	90
Tomato and Cheese ☐	½ cup packed	12	95
and Cucumber ☐	3 oz.	11	110
stuffed ☐	1 small used	9	75
Tossed ☐	1 cup packed	10	35
with French Dressing ☐	1 tbs.	20	135
Tomato and Cucumber ☐	3 oz.	12	90
Tomato Aspic ☐	½ cup	20	100
Tuna ☐	4 tbs. used	10	110
Vegetable Combination ☐	½ cup	25	40
Waldorf ☐	½ cup packed	40	145

Salad Dressings

ITEM	PORTION	CARBO-CALS	CALORIES
Bacon and Vingear ☐	2 tbs.	4	58
Bleu Cheese ☐	1 tbs.	4	100
Boiled Dressing ☐	1 tbs.	12	28
French Dressing ☐	1 tbs.	4	100
Diet ☐	1 tbs.	4	25
Commercial ☐	1 tbs.	12	65
Homemade ☐	1 tbs.	4	100
Fruit Gelatin Dressing ☐	1 tbs.	10	22
Home Cooked Salad Dressing ☐	1 tbs.	8	42
Mayonnaise ☐	1 tbs.	trace	100
with mineral oil ☐		trace	100
Commercial Dressing ☐	1 tbs.	trace	108
Diet Dressing ☐	1 tbs.	trace	35
Miracle Whip ☐	1 tbs.	trace	52

ITEM	PORTION	CARBO-CALS	CALORIES
Oils, Salad or			
Cooking ○	1 tbs.	0	124
Olive Oil ○	1 tbs.	0	110
Peanut Oil ○	1 tbs.	0	108
Roquefort Dressing ○	1 tbs.	trace	100
Russian Dressing □	1 tbs.	4	106
Thousand Island			
Dressing □	1 tbs.	4	100
Diet ○	1 tbs.	trace	50
Vinegar ○	1 tbs.	trace	2
Vinegar and oil ½			
and ½ ○	1 tbs.	trace	51
Vinegar and Bacon ○	2 tbs.	trace	58

Sandwiches

(MADE WITH TWO SLICES OF BREAD)

ITEM	PORTION	CARBO-CALS	CALORIES
American Cheese +	2 med. slices used	125	330
Bacon and Egg +	2 med. slices & 1 egg	130	327
Bacon and Lettuce +	2 slices ea. used	130	232
Bacon and Tomato			
and Lettuce +	2 slices used	120	235
Barbecue Beef +	2 oz. beef used	96	250
Barbecue Pork +	2 oz. pork used	96	310
Bologna +	2 slices used	100	360
Calves Liver +	3 oz. used	120	250
Camembert Cheese +	1 triangle used	100	215
Cevelat +	2 slices	100	230
Chateau Cheese +	2 oz. pc.	115	330
Cheddar Cheese +	2 oz. used	104	356
Cheese and Olive +	1	100	350
Cheeseburger +	1	100	500
Chicken Liver +	3 oz. used	100	285
Chicken salad +	3 oz. used	100	210
Chicken, Sliced +	2 slices	100	205
with gravy +		180	398
Club +	3 decker	165	575
Corned Beef +	2 oz. beef used	96	250
Crabmeat +	4 oz. meat used	102	280

ITEM	PORTION	CARBO-CALS	CALORIES
Cream Cheese +	2 oz. used	100	342
and Nut +		110	400
and Jelly +		200	442
and Olives +		120	392
Denver, Western +	1 med. egg used	118	400
Egg, Fried +	1 med. egg used	100	230
Egg Salad +	1 med. egg used	100	265
Frankfurter +	1 med. used	88	254
Ham +			
Baked +	1 lg. slice	98	395
Boiled +	3 oz. sliced	98	468
Fried +	3 oz. slice	96	472
Luncheon Meat +	3 oz. sliced	100	388
and Swiss Cheese +	3 oz ham		
	1 oz. cheese	100	538
Ham Salad +	3 oz. used	120	474
Hamburger +	1½ oz. gr. beef	100	288
Lettuce and Tomato +	1 tomato and 4 leaves		
	of lettuce	104	167
Liverwurst +	2 slices	100	430
Meat Loaf +	1 lg. slice	140	450
Oyster, Fried +	1 lg. used	160	242
Pastrami +	2 med. slices used	96	300
Peanut Butter +	2 tbs. used	120	330
with Jelly +		140	500
Pimento Cheese +	2 oz. used	110	334
Pork Chop +	1 chop used	120	423
Pork Sausage +	4 oz. used	110	470
Roast Beef +	2 oz. beef used	120	310
with gravy +		150	420
Roast Pork +	3 oz. used	120	414
with gravy +		150	510
Roquefort +	2 oz. used	110	304
Cheese spread +		115	334
Salami +	2 slices used	110	360
Salmon +		110	350
Salmon Salad +	3 oz. used	120	370
Sardine +	3 oz. used	110	358
Shrimp Salad +	1 sandwich	110	200
Shrimp, Fried +	6 medium used	160	230
Sole, Fillet of +	4 oz. fish	150	208

ITEM	PORTION	CARBO-CALS	CALORIES
Steak +	1 sandwich	115	300
Summer Sausage +	2 slices ¼" thick	120	230
Swiss Cheese +	3 oz. sliced	125	445
Tongue +	4 oz. sliced	120	365
Tuna +	3 oz. used	120	280
Tuna Salad +	4 oz. used	125	330
Turkey +	4 oz. sliced	120	448
with gravy +		150	600
Vienna Sausage +	4 oz. used	120	374

Sauces

ITEM	PORTION	CARBO-CALS	CALORIES
A-1 Sauce ☐	1 tbs.	9	25
Barbecue ☐	1 tbs.	32	40
Butterscotch ☐	1 tbs.	24	35
Caramel +	¼ cup	240	270
Catsup, Tomato ☐	1 tbs.	16	17
Cheese ☐	¼ cup	20	130
Cherry Sauce ☐	1 tbs.	20	25
Chili Sauce ☐	1 tbs.	16	17
Chocolate ☐	1 tbs.	8	100
Cranberry ☐	2 tbs.	70	88
Cream Sauce ☐	3 oz.	30	350
Creole Sauce ☐	¼ cup	32	100
Fudge +	¼ cup	280	360
Garlic Sauce ☐			
with butter ☐	1 tbs.	2	100
with water ☐	1 tbs.	0	0
Gravy, thick +	1 tbs.	40	50
thin ☐	1 tbs.	30	35
Hard Sauce ☐	1 tbs.	24	45
Hollandaise Sauce ☐	1 tbs.	trace	65
Mock ☐	1 tbs.	4	75
Lemon ☐	1 tbs.	28	30
Marshmallow +	¼ cup	100	110
Meat Sauce, Italian ☐	¼ cup	80	115
Mustard ☐	2 tbs.	4	35
Plum Pudding Sauce +	1 tbs.	70	97
Raisin +	2 tbs.	95	100
Simple Sugar +	1 tbs.	100	100

ITEM	PORTION	CARBO-CALS	CALORIES
Sour Cream ☐	2 tbs.	28	112
Soya Sauce ☐	1 tbs.	5	7
Tartar Sauce ☐	1 tbs.	4	100
Tomato Sauce ☐	½ cup	28	100
White Sauce ☐	½ cup	30	190
Wine Sauce ☐	1 tbs.	18	20
Worcestershire Sauce ☐	1 tbs.	12	24

Soups

ITEM	PORTION	CARBO-CALS	CALORIES
Asparagus, Creamed ☐	8 oz. cup	64	201
Barley ☐	8 oz. cup	56	117
Bean, Navy +	8 oz. cup	108	200
Beef Broth ☐	8 oz. cup	20	70
Beef Creamed ☐	8 oz. cup	50	205
Beef Noodle ☐	1 serving	28	100
Beef with Vegetable and Barley ☐	1 serving	35	120
Bouillon, Clear ○	8 oz. cup	trace	9
cube ○	1	trace	2
Celery, Creamed ☐	8 oz. cup	52	201
Chicken			
Broth ○	8 oz. cup	0	50
Creamed ☐	8 oz. cup	20	200
Gumbo ☐	8 oz. cup	50	155
Infant Food ☐	1 oz. strained	trace	17
and Matzoth Balls ☐	2 balls and 1 cup	60	200
Noodle ☐	8 oz. cup	28	100
and Rice ☐	8 oz. cup	18	100
Vegetable ☐	8 oz. cup	30	90
Chili Beef Soup +	1 serving	75	200
Clam Chowder ☐			
with milk ☐	1 serving	28	100
with tomato ☐	1 serving	32	120
Consomme, Clear ○	8 oz. cup	0	5
Corn Chowder, Creamed +	8 oz. cup	70	198
Creamed Soups (most) ☐	8 oz. cup	40	180

ITEM	PORTION	CARBO-CALS	CALORIES
Duck, Creamed ☐	8 oz. cup	40	200
Green Pea +	1 serving	90	150
with ham +	1 serving	100	180
Gumbo Creole ☐	8 oz. cup	40	100
Jellied Consomme ○	1 serving	0	10
Lentil +	8 oz. cup	200	600
Mock Turtle ☐	8 oz. cup	50	109
Mullegatawny ☐	8 oz. cup		165
Mushroom, Creamed ☐	8 oz. cup	40	195
Noodle ☐	8 oz. cup	28	100
Onion ☐			
Creamed ☐	8 oz. cup	28	200
French ☐	8 oz. cup	35	150
Oxtail ☐	8 oz. cup	35	150
Oyster Stew ½ cream,			
½ milk +	8 oz. cup	100	200
whole milk +	8 oz. cup	120	244
skimmed milk +	8 oz. cup	140	155
Pea +	8 oz. cup	100	200
Creamed +	8 oz. cup	80	225
Pepperpot ☐	8 oz. cup	35	175
Potato +	8 oz. cup	100	185
Creamed +	8 oz. cup	75	215
Rice +	8 oz. cup	70	117
Scotch Broth ☐	8 oz. cup	36	100
Shrimp, Creamed ☐	1 serving	44	120
Spinach ☐	8 oz. cup	44	205
Split Pea +	8 oz. cup	96	210
Creamed +	8 oz. cup	100	265
Tomato, Clear +	8 oz. cup	80	75
Creamed +	8 oz. cup	80	202
Rice +	1 serving	85	210
Vegetable ☐	1 serving	50	180
Turkey Noodle ☐	1 serving	28	100
Vegetable ☐	8 oz. cup	30	82
and Lamb, Infant ○	1 oz. strained	trace	14
and Beef ☐	8 oz. cup	50	182
Infant, ☐	1 oz. strained	trace	12
Creamed ☐	8 oz. cup	40	220
Vichyssoise ☐	1 serving	48	200

ITEM	PORTION	CARBO-CALS	CALORIES
	Sugars		
Beet Sugar +	1 tbs.	45	45
Brown Sugar (packed) +	1 tbs.	50	51
Brown Sugar (packed) +	8 oz. cup	813	813
Cane Sugar +	1 tbs.	45	45
Cube Sugar +	1 lump	27	27
Dextro Maltose +	1 tbs.	40	40
Granulated Sugar +	1 tbs.	45	45
Maple Sugar +	3½ oz.	360	360
Powdered Sugar +	1 tbs.	30	30
	Sweets		
Almonds, Chocolate Covered +	6	34	160
Almond Joy +	10 cent bar	88	218
Bar, Average +	2 oz. - 5 cent bar	80	275
Bonbons +	1 round pc.	36	75
Brown Sugar Fudge +	1 pc.	88	200
Butterscotch +	1 square pc.	16	75
Candy, Bar, Avg. +	2 oz. - 5 cent bar	80	275
Candy, Hard +	1 oz.	100	110
Caramels, Plain +	1 square pc. - 1 oz.	88	120
with nuts +		90	130
Cherries, Candied +	1 square pc.	40	125
Chocolate Bar, Plain +	2 oz. - 5 cent bar	128	300
with nuts +	2 oz. - 5 cent bar	136	350
Bitter, Plain +	1 oz. bar	35	140
Semi-Sweet +	1 oz.	68	145
Milk +	1 oz.	62	155
with almonds +	1 oz.	66	170
Sweet +	1 oz. square	72	180
with almonds +	1 oz. square	68	220
Chocolate Creams +	1 oz. piece	80	110
Chocolate Fudge +	1 oz. piece	92	115
Chocolate Kisses +	5 css. - 1 oz.		100

ITEM	PORTION	CARBO-CALS	CALORIES
Chocolate Mints,			
Cream +	1 oz. pc.	90	110
	5 cent size	92	150
	3 small	88	130
Citron Candy +	1 oz. pc.	80	90
Clark Bar +	5 cent bar	84	126
Cocoanut Creams +	1 square pc.	80	100
Cough Drops +	1 average pc.	8	10
Date Creams +	1 oz. pc.	80	115
Dates, Pitted +	1 oz. pc.	30	40
Stuffed, nuts +	1 oz. pc.	35	48
unpitted +	1 oz. pc.	25	32
Divinity Fudge +	1 oz. pc.	88	115
Fifth Avenue +	5 cent bar	70	116
Fondant Candy +	1 oz. pc.	40	105
Fruit Drops +	3 medium pcs.	40	100
Fudge Chocolate +	1 oz. square	100	115
with nuts +	1 oz. square	72	120
Ginger Root,			
Crystallized +	1 oz. pc.	90	97
Glazed Fruit +	1 oz. pc.	32	95
Grapefruit Peel Candy +	1 oz. pc.	80	90
Gum +	1 stick	7	9
Candy Coated +	2 average pcs.	10	13
Gum Drops +	1 lg. pc.	30	35
	8 sm. pcs.	35	40
Halvah +	1⅛ oz. pc.	90	116
Hard Candy +	1 oz.	100	110
Hershey Milk			
Chocolate +	Plain, 5 cent bar	65	115
with almonds +	5 cent bar	65	120
Jelly Beans +	6 pcs.	40	50
Lemon Drops +	' round pc.	12	15
Lemon Peel Candy +	1 oz. pc.	80	90
Life Savers +	1 pc. with hole	4	5
	1 pc. without hole	8	10
Maple Sugar +	1 medium pc.	80	105
Mars Candy Bar +	5 cent bar	80	168
Mars,			
Forever Yours +	5 cent bar	80	140
Mars, Milky Way +	5 cent bar	100	138

ITEM	PORTION	CARBO-CALS	CALORIES
Mars, Snickers +	5 cent bar	100	135
Mars, Three Musketeers +	5 cent bar	100	165
Marshmallows +			
Chocolate +	1 pc.	32	105
Plain +	1 pc.	24	90
Afterdinner, chocolate +	1 small	45	90
Afterdinner, chocolate +	1 medium	50	110
Plain +	5 small	6	50
Cream +	2 small	10	60
Molasses Kisses +	1 average pc.	20	25
Mounds +	10 cent bar	200	238
Nestle's			
Milk Chocoate +	5 cent plain bar	60	115
with almonds +	5 cent bar	60	105
Crunch +	5 cent bar	60	107
Nougats +			
Plain +	1 oz. pc.	65	115
with nuts +	1 oz. pc.	65	125
Oh Henry +	5 cent bar	85	142
Orange Drops +	1 round pc.	12	15
Orange Peel Candy +	1 oz. pc.	85	90
Peanut Bar, average +	5 cent bar	80	260
Peanut Brittle +	1 oz. pc.	80	125
Peppermint Patty, Chocolate Covered +	1 medium pc.	60	90
Peppermint Stick +	1 oz. pc.	70	95
Powerhouse +	5 cent bar	80	116
Praline +	3" diameter pc.	100	300
Sour Balls, Hard +	1 average pc.	18	20
Taffy +			
Salt Water +	1 average kiss	25	50
Turkish +	1 average kiss	25	35
	5 cent bar	60	140
Toffee +			
Coffee +	1 sm. pc.	18	20
English +	1 sm. pc.	20	25
Tootsie Roll +	5 cent roll	60	110

ITEM	PORTION	CARBO-CALS	CALORIES
Turkish Delight +	1" sq. pc.	18	20
Turkish Taffy +	5 cent bar	80	140

Syrups

ITEM	PORTION	CARBO-CALS	CALORIES
Cane Sugar Syrup +	⅓ cup	300	300
Chocolate +	⅓ cup	252	250
Corn +	⅓ cup	300	300
Honey +	5 tbs.	320	320
Maple, Pure +	5 tbs.	256	256
Molasses, Cane +	5 tbs.	285	285
Syrups (Most table blends) +	1 tbs.	57	57

Vegetables

ITEM	PORTION	CARBO-CALS	CALORIES
Ameranth ☐	3½ oz.	30	36
Arrowhead ☐	3½ oz. of tubers	52	106
Arrowroot +	3½ oz.	100	126
Artichoke ☐			
Hearts, canned ☐	5	32	37
French +	1	80	120
Jerusalem ☐	4 small	68	78
Bottom ☐	1	20	30
Asparagus ☐			
Stalks, Cooked ☐	6	12	22
cut spears ☐	¾ cup	14	30
Canned,			
cut spears ☐	1 cup	24	43
Canned ☐	6 spears	12	22
Frozen ☐	6 spears	12	22
cut spears ☐	1 cup	20	36
Aster Leaves ☐	3½ oz. portion	20	31
Balsampear ☐	3½ oz.	10	29
Bamboo Shoots ☐	3½ oz.	22	27
Beans			
Baked, Canned, pork and molasses +	1 cup	200	325
Baked, Canned,			

ITEM	PORTION	CARBO-CALS	CALORIES
tomato sauce +	1 cup	180	295
Green, cooked ☐	1 cup	12	27
Green, canned ☐	¾ cup	30	50
Green, canned ☐	1 cup w/liquid	24	43
Green, strained ☐	1 oz.	4	6
Kidney +	7 tbs.	64	180
Lima +	½ cup cooked	100	130
Lima, canned +	1 cup	120	176
Lima, frozen +	3½ oz.	68	130
Bean Sprouts			
Mung ☐	1 cup	16	27
Soy ☐	1 cup	20	30
Beet Greens ☐	½ cup cooked	20	39
Beets			
Raw ☐	2 medium	40	104
Cooked ☐	½ cup	44	55
Canned ☐	½ cup	44	60
Canned, strained ☐	1 oz.	8	10
Pickled ☐	1 cup	44	56
Broccoli ☐			
Cooked ☐	1 cup	32	44
Frozen ☐	2 - 3 spears	16	20
Brussel Sprouts,			
Cooked ☐	1 cup	32	44
Burdock Root +	3½ oz. portion	60	94
Cabbage			
Shredded ☐	1 cup	20	24
Chinese ☐	1 cup	8	14
Chinese, Cooked ☐	1 cup	16	27
1 wedge ☐		8	24
Calabash ☐	3½ oz.	8	17
Carrots ☐			
Raw ☐	1	20	21
Raw, Grated ☐	1 cup	40	45
Cooked ☐	1 cup diced	36	44
Canned ☐	1 cup diced	40	44
Canned, strained ☐	1 oz.	6	7
Cauliflower ☐			
Buds, ☐	1 cup	20	25
Cooked ☐	1 cup	24	30
Frozen ☐	1 cup	28	35

ITEM	PORTION	CARBO-CALS	CALORIES
Cedar Leaves ☐	3½ oz.	20	45
Celeriac ☐	4 - 6 roots	32	45
	8 - 14 roots	60	90
Celery ☐	1 lg. stalk	6	7
Diced ☐	1 cup	15	18
Cooked ☐	1 cup	18	24
Fresh ☐	3 small inner stalks	6	9
Chard ☐	1 cup cooked leaves	8	47
Leaves and Stalks ☐	1 cup cooked	25	30
Chayote ☐	3½ oz.	8	28
Chives, chopped ☐	3½ oz.	8	42
Chicory ☐	5 or 6 leaves	16	18
Chrysanthemum ☐	3½ oz.	12	17
Collards ☐	1 cup	52	76
Coriander ☐	3½ oz.	80	140
Corn +	1 ear	120	150
	1 cup kernels	115	140
Canned, w/liquid +	1 cup	160	170
Corn Fritter +	1	40	50
Cowpeas +	1 cup cooked	100	151
Cress ☐			
Garden ☐	1 lb.	60	186
Garden ☐	1 cup cooked	40	73
Water ☐	1 lb.	60	180
Water ☐	1 bunch	20	40
Water ☐	10 sprigs	1	2
Cucumber ☐	1 medium	6	12
Dandelion Greens ☐	¾ cup cooked	52	75
Egg Plant ☐	½ cup	15	52
Endive ☐	10 leaves	4	6
Escarole ☐	2 lg. leaves	4	6
Fennel ☐	1 cup	8	12
Garlic ☐	1 clove	4	5
Ginger Root ☐	3½ oz.	28	51
Hominy Grits +	½ cup cooked	52	65
Horse-radish ☐	1 tbs.	10	12
Kale ☐	½ cup cooked	32	55
Kohlrabi, cooked, fresh +	8 oz. cup sliced	52	72
Leeks ☐	3 medium	18	42
Lentils +	¾ cup	140	315

ITEM	PORTION	CARBO-CALS	CALORIES
Lettuce ☐	1 compact head	18	68
Lotus Root +	⅔ average segment	40	49
Matai, Fresh +	3½ oz.	50	78
Mint ☐	1 tsp. chopped	0	8
Mushrooms ☐	4 large	3	4
canned, 1 cup with			
liquid ☐		15	28
Sauteed ☐	7 small	10	60
Fresh ☐	8 oz. cup sliced	12	20
Button ☐	3½ oz.	8	16
Mustard, Dry ☐	1 tsp.	0	10
Mustard Greens ☐	1 cup cooked	20	31
Okra ☐	¼ cup	12	19
Olives ☐			
Green ☐	10 large	4	104
Ripe or Black ☐	10 large	8	135
Stuffed ☐	5 mammoth	7	55
Onions			
Raw ☐	1 medium	40	49
	1 tbs. chopped	3	4
Cooked ☐	1 cup	72	79
Green ☐	6 small	20	23
Scalloped ☐	½ cup	60	70
Fried ☐	½ cup	140	162
Spanish ☐	1 medium size	6	8
Creamed ☐	½ cup	80	108
Stewed ☐	½ cup	40	50
Oyster Plant ☐	½ cup cooked	28	35
Parsley ☐	1 tbs. chopped	trace	1
Parsnips +	½ cup cooked	40	47
Raw +	3½ oz.	65	78
Peas +			
Fresh, Cooked +	1 cup	80	111
Fresh, Cooked +	1 lb. in pod	144	316
Canned, with liquid +	1 cup	132	168
Canned, Drained +	1 cup	112	145
Canned, strained +	1 oz.	8	14
Frozen +	½ cup	44	
Split, cooked +	1 cup	140	
Fresh, Garden, Shelled +	3½ oz.	75	90

ITEM	PORTION	CARBO-CALS	CALORIES
Peppers ☐			
Green ☐	1 medium	12	16
Green, Stuffed ☐	1 medium	48	185
Red, Hot Dried ☐	1 tbs.	36	52
Red ☐	1 medium	16	28
Cooked ☐	1 medium	12	17
Pickle			
Chow Chow ☐	4 pcs.	4	7
Cucumber, Bread			
& Butter ☐	4 slices	18	20
Dill ☐	1 medium	12	15
Sweet ☐	1 large	10	22
Sour ☐	1 large	12	15
Sweet Mixed Relish ☐	1 tbs.	12	14
with mustard ☐	1 tbs.	14	16
Pimento ☐	1 medium canned	8	10
Potato Chips +	10	40	108
Potatoes			
Au Gratin +	4 oz.	48	250
Baked or Boiled +	1 medium	80	100
Canned +	3 - 4 small	75	90
Creamed +	½ cup	56	125
French fried +	10 pcs.	80	157
Hash Brown +	1 cup	240	470
French Fried,			
frozen +	10 pcs.	60	148
Fried +	½ cup	120	239
Mashed, with milk +	½ cup	60	79
Mashed, with			
butter +	½ cup	52	120
Baked with peel +	1 medium	80	102
Baked without peel +	1 medium	70	97
Boiled, peeled +	1 medium	75	105
Boiled, peeled +	8 oz. cup	75	105
Boiled, unpeeled +	1 medium	80	181
Boiled, unpeeled +	1 lb.	150	359
Canned, drained +	3 - 4 small	80	118
Canned, drained +	1 lb.	150	378
Mashed +	1 cup	90	240
Pressure Cooked +	1 medium	75	105
Pressure Cooked +	1 cup diced	75	105

ITEM	PORTION	CARBO-CALS	CALORIES
Steamed +	1 medium	75	105
Steamed +	1 cup diced	75	105
Scalloped +	½ cup	60	121
Pumpkin +	3½ oz.	28	31
Canned +	1 cup	70	76
Radishes ☐	4 small	4	7
Chinese Radishes ☐	3½ oz.	16	19
Rice			
Converted and Cooked +	8 oz. cup	160	204
Fried +	8 oz. cup	160	258
Pre-Cooked Dry +	8 oz. cup	180	420
Spanish +	8 oz. cup	140	300
White, Boiled +	8 oz. cup	160	201
Wild Rice +	8 oz. cup	180	240
Romaine ☐	¼ head	3	4
Rutabaga ☐	1 cup cooked	50	60
Sauerkraut ☐	½ cup drained	20	27
Scallions ☐	4 medium	4	8
Sesame Seeds ☐	1 oz.	0	8
Shepherdspurse ☐	3½ oz.	25	39
Sorrel ☐	4 oz. cup	trace	5
Soy Beans ☐			
Fresh ☐	½ cup	trace	119
Soybean Sprouts ☐	1 cup	24	60
Snow Peas ☐	14	20	30
Spinach ☐			
Raw ☐	½ pound	24	44
Cooked ☐	1 cup	24	46
Canned ☐	1 cup	24	46
Canned, Strained ☐	1 oz.	3	5
Tomatoes ☐			
Canned ☐	8 oz. cup	9	46
Fresh ☐	1 medium	6	30
Fresh ☐	1 small	4	22
Stewed ☐	8 oz. cup	9	50
Puree, Canned ☐	1 cup	18	
Squash			
Hubbard or Winter, Baked +	½ cup	44	50

ITEM	PORTION	CARBO-CALS	CALORIES
Hubbard or Winter, frozen +	1 cup boiled	40	45
Summer, Boiled ☐	½ cup	16	19
Summer, Canned Strained ☐	1 oz.	4	8
Hubbard +	½ cup	44	50
Winter, Baked or Mashed +	1 cup	80	97
Winter, Boiled and Mashed +	1 cup	80	86
String Beans, fresh ☐	6 tbs.	16	21
Succotash + Canned +	½ cup	60	68
Swamp Cabbage ☐	3½ oz.	15	29
Sweet Potatoes + Raw +	3½ oz.	100	123
Baked +	1	140	183
Boiled +	1	160	252
Candied +	1 small	240	314
Canned +	1 cup	216	233
Boiled +	1 lb.	330	560
Turnip Tops ☐	½ cup cooked	28	49
Turnips Cooked ☐	½ cup	16	22
Mashed ☐	8 oz. cup	45	60
Water cress ☐	10 pcs.	1	2
Yams Cooked +	1 cup	180	260
Baked, peeled +	1	160	183
Boiled, peeled +	1	170	252
Candied +	1 small	220	314
Yautia ☐	½ of 4" long piece	28	75
Zucchini ☐	½ cup	16	23

5

Eating Well
To . . .

They say that the first day of any diet is the hardest, because by the second day you are not on it any more. This could not be farther from the truth when you substitute proteins for carbohydrates, because eating well becomes as zealously guarded a habit with you as eating sweets. Columnist Earl Wilson went from 153 pounds to 138 during the first month that he traded carbohydrates for proteins. The 15 pound loss, he says, made him look ten years younger.

Have you checked your scale in the past few days? If you have started to trade carbohydrates for proteins in your shopping and

. . . Lose Weight

on your menus, you have started to lose weight. Because the transition has out of common sense been a gradual one, the weight loss may be imperceptible at first. But if you are the average person, the day you complete your transition to 250 carbo-cals is the day you will lose your first "pound of flesh" and from then on watch them melt away.

Losing physical mass seems to have properties of inertia and momentum that we find in the science of matter. You have to push extra hard to get something started. Once it is sliding or rolling, it is easier to keep it going. Inertia, reinforced by something called starting friction, needs to be overcome at the outset.

Most physicians place the overweight person on a 1,000 to 1,200 total calorie diet to start the reducing process. This is a giant step—less than half of the 2,500 to 3,000 calories that the person has probably been consuming daily up until then. One pound is equivalent to 3,500 calories. One would think that cutting down 500 calories for seven days, a total loss of 3,500 calories, would produce a pound or more of weight loss. But don't bet on it!

There might very well be an inertia about the body's conversion of its own fat to energy, but there appears to be a more obvious answer—carbohydrates. Assuming that the average reducing diet is about 40% to 50% carbohydrate, were a physician to cut your total food intake in half and to prescribe 1,500 total calories, the carbohydrate level would still be above 600 calories. This may not be a fattening amount, but it is most certainly not enough of a cut for most people to lose any significant amount of weight. When the total diet is cut to 1,000 or 1,200 calories, only then does the carbohydrate calorie count coincidentally drop below the probable 400-500 count needed to lose weight. The protein and fat intake could be even higher and the same weight loss would result.

What, all that starvation for nought? Just about. If the carbo-cals alone are cut, the same weight loss is possible—without the starvation symptoms and shock to the system. This is the whole secret to happy, healthful slenderizing. This is the process for which you have set the stage and are ready to begin.

Prepare A Progress Chart

There is no "if" about your losing weight now. Just "how much" and "how fast." Now is the time for scientific observation and controls. Like a balloonist, you have dropped carbohydrate ballast to get lighter. If you lighten too fast, a corrective adjustment—as simple as a slice of bread—may be needed. Once you lighten your body weight all you want, a similar adjustment is needed to halt the process. If you do not lose weight fast enough, more carbohydrates may have to go.

A line graph is a simple way to portray your weight loss. If the line slants upward, you are gaining; if it stays horizontal, you are not changing; if it slants downward, you are losing. The line also clearly depicts your rate of loss. It may start down steeply as your weight loss begins, and then the slope may become less steep as your rate of weight loss slows up. It may even have peaks and valleys as temporary interruptions and setbacks occur.

Here is how to make the chart you need for your line graph. A piece of cross-sectional graph paper will save you time. Otherwise take an ordinary piece of white paper. Place it in front of you so that its long dimension is horizontal. Draw a heavy line nearly top to bottom on the left side. This is your vertical axis. It will record the pounds. Now from the bottom of this axis draw a heavy horizontal line from left to right across the page. This is your horizontal axis. It will record the days. Now at quarter inch intervals draw light horizontal lines and at the same quarter inch intervals draw vertical lines. Each horizontal line is a pound. Each vertical line is a day.

At the top of your vertical axis place a heavy dot. To the left of it write in your weight today. Then write a column of figures extending down the axis one pound less for each line down. Write a series of dates below the horizontal axis progress one day for each line across.

If you used an average size piece of paper 8½ by 11 inches, your weights will extend from your present weight down to a weight loss of 30 pounds or so. If you do not expect to lose this much, decide on a goal and then draw a heavy horizontal line at this weight. Mark it "goal."

In a couple of days you will weigh yourself again and place a dot where the right date line and weight line meet. You will then connect it with the dot you made today and you will have started your progress chart. Note that there is no room on the chart to record a weight gain after today. An oversight? No indeed, your weight now goes only in one unmistakable direction—down!

The Scale And You

If you own a small bathroom floor scale, see that it is adjusted so that it reaches zero when not in use. Always use it in the same spot. A scale can read one or two pounds up or down if carried to a different part of the house, due to slight variations in floor level. Never place such a scale on a soft carpeted surface, as this can cause wide inaccuracy.

Another cause of inaccuracy can be the way you stand on a scale. Stand naturally and erect. Lower your head just enough to read the result. If you lean forward, many floor scales will falsely read more. If you lean backward, they read falsely less. (Lean backward in cutting your carbohydrates and the scale will truly read less.) Standing slightly forward or back of center on the scale's platform can cause the same inaccuracy, so note where your toes are and try to stand the same way each time.

To obtain further accuracy in weighing yourself, try to be in the same state of dress or undress when you weigh yourself, and stick to the same time of the day. A person can weigh one or two pounds more after dinner than before breakfast, and a trip to the bathroom can make a difference. An accurate progress chart will be a helpful adjunct to you in the reducing days ahead.

Daily weighing is not necessary. In fact, there are advantages in limiting your trips to the scale at most to twice a week. It can be discouraging to see only a very minute change. A steady daily loss at the rate of 10 pounds a month (⅓ pound a day) would hardly show on the common floor scale.

Furthermore there are day-to-day physiological changes in the human body which affect weight temporarily. The amount of spice in the food you eat can affect the body's tendency to hold water. Salt can do the same. A hot humid day can cause a loss of body fluid. Women often build up several pounds of water prior to the menstrual cycle. Men can lose a pound or more at a tense, drawn out meeting.

Each time you weigh yourself place a dot opposite the proper date and weight on your progress chart and draw a line to connect it with the previous dot. The resulting weight loss graph will tell you at a glance how well your high protein fare is faring.

Carbo-cal Countdown

The countdown is now under way. All preparations have been made. The kitchen is well stocked with high protein foods. You have analyzed your eating habits and found high protein substitutes for high carbohydrate fatteners. You have planned some tantalizing dishes for the days ahead. You have already started to switch some carbohydrate foods in favor of protein foods. You are acquainted with carbo-cals and how to count them, using the tables in the recipe section. You are ready to start your first day at the 250 carbo-cal level.

The first day is not a day of deprivation or wistful longing, of hunger pangs or dizzy spells. It is a day you will be eating more nourishingly than you probably have been doing in the past, a day when you will be bending the elbow before lunch and dinner if that is your pleasure. Your friends will notice one difference: You will be making frequent reference to your carbo-cal tables and jotting down little columns of figures. They might also notice that you use an artificial sweetener in your coffee, that you order a rasher of bacon instead of your usual toasted English muffin, and that you switched from whiskey sours to vodka martinis.

The major effort in this final count-down phase comes in trimming the carbohydrate values that sneak in the back door, so to speak—the hard candies, chewing gum, fruit snacks and beverages that find their way to use during the average day. These are more like social habits rather than eating habits. They are not usually founded on hunger or any basic need of the body. We might acquire them because they provide a feeling of belonging, or they free us of self-consciousness, or they give us a sense of security.

Taken in any quantity, these extraordinary carbo-cals encroach on our 250 carbo-cal budget, replacing nourishing food like fruit juices and vegetables which provide us with essential nutrients. Some day our candy counters may see an assortment of chewing gum and candies made of nutrients and concentrates on the protein side, so that we can obtain essential food while engaging in our habit of oral manipulation.

Meanwhile, we must cut down, replace, and do without. We must use artificial sweeteners and non-caloric or diet brands. We might even try water instead of sugary soda pop. One man who was an inveterate gum chewer now carries a piece of modeling clay with him at all times. No, he does not chew it, he uses it as a fingering piece. He throws it up and lets it hit his palm with a resounding slap, squeezes it and fingers it as he talks. You could not get him to chew another stick of gum.

It is of top priority that every time we do place something in our mouth, we add its carbo-cals to our total. We must not exceed our 250 limit. For some people 50 carbo-cals over cancels it altogether and 250 carbo-cals over can reverse it to weight gain. Take the case of Helen:

CASE HISTORY G-20

Her Weight Was A Headache

Helen, 19, was referred by her physician to my office. Besides being 20 pounds overweight at 141, she suffered from severe migraine-type headaches and had high blood pressure to boot. She had been on a 1000-calorie reducing diet for four weeks and the scale had not budged.

I had her make an accurate record for one week of everything she was consuming right down to even the water she drank. The record showed she was eating reasonably well at the table, but in between sittings were such items as a coke, and as many as three rolls of hard candy a day. At 35 carbo-cals in each package and additional carbo-cals in the soft drinks, Helen's carbo-cal intake was actually 800 per day!

By adding more meat, fish, cheese and eggs to her regular meals and cutting carbo-cals to 200 per day, Helen's weight began to drop. She was no longer starved between meals and her desire for the cokes and hard candies ceased. In nine weeks she lost 20 pounds. Her high blood pressure also went down. Her headaches must have had something to do with her high blood pressure or tension over her excessive weight or both because they, too, are gone.

There is no borrowing from tomorrow's quota. Overdrawing your account by 100 carbo-cals today does not mean that you can recoup by cutting out 100 carbo-cals starting with breakfast to-morrow. First, the excess carbo-cals will already have done their fattening work, providing not just the fat they turn into them-selves but also helping to convert some of the day's protein and fat to additional fat.

Secondly, tomorrow's quota cannot rightly be cut 100 carbo-cals. The 250 carbo-cal quota is close to your daily minimum re-quirement. Cutting it down to repent for yesterday invites low-ered resistance that comes with improper nutrition.

Solve today's problems today. Fortunately there are a number of situations, not one of which is starvation or even doing without. All you need to do is find something you like that is high in pro-tein to substitute for something you like that is high in carbo-hydrate.

Go, Caution, And Stop Foods

The list that starts on page 110 provides you with a quick way to select low-carbohydrate foods. Each food is identified with a symbol as follows:

O This is a GO food, little or no carbo-cals.

☐ This food contains a moderate amount of carbo-cals, but use CAUTION in including them in your meals.

+ This is classified as a STOP food because it is heavy in carbo-cals. STOP foods are detrimental to your program of weight control.

As to "GO" foods, tagged with symbol "O," you can literally eat all you want of these nourishing foods. These are the substitutes that you use to replace the foods that are further down on the list and higher in carbo-cals.

As to "CAUTION" foods, tagged with symbol "☐", here is where your serious counting must be carried out. There is usually no need to seek substitutes for "caution" foods, but you cannot eat all you want of "caution" foods or you will find your menu for the day thrown out of kilter by such a run on carbohydrates.

"STOP" foods, tagged with symbol "+", are usually so high in carbo-cals as to be prohibitive. A substitute is almost always mandatory.

There is nothing your body needs in the "stop" foods that is not supplied in the "caution" and "go" foods. A diversified menu of "caution" and "go" is a healthful, nutritious menu. You can kiss "stop" foods goodbye permanently; if you can educate your taste buds not to miss them; your body most certainly will never miss them. If you must indulge, shuffle your menu to keep the carbo-cals total below 250 and keep the portion down to a bare minimum. But wouldn't you prefer a filet mignon?

Two criticisms have been leveled against low carbohydrate diets, which are really not valid criticisms of the diet but of the dieter. The first criticism says that *it is a "quickie" diet and does not achieve permanent weight control.* In actuality, it is the only permanent way to weight control because it is not a diet at all. It is a return to normalcy. However, the dieter can make it a "quickie" by not seeking substitutes so much more delicious and satisfying than what they are replacing that they become permanent. This requires planning and ingenuity at the start—but then there will never be a finish.

A second common criticism of the low carbohydrate diet is that *it is not a nutritious diet.* This is true only when the dieter prefers "stop" sweets to "caution" fruits and vegetables. Let the dieter substitute tasty wholesome protein foods for decadent sickly sweet foods and he is sure to be on a higher level of nutrition. In fact, he will be on an even higher level of nutrition than most diets that starve the body on a 1,000 to 1,200 calorie regimen, for there will be more protein and more vitamins and minerals simply because there is more of the same food (except fattening carbohydrate).

The Recommended Dietary Allowances of the Food and Nutrition Board of the National Research Council prescribes 2,200 to 2,900 total calories for U. S. men depending on weight, age and height, and 1,600 to 2,100 total calories for U. S. women. The only diet that can provide this many calories and still deliver a weight loss is a low carbohydrate diet.

The Board also recommends at least 350 protein calories for men and at least 290 for women, but makes no recommendation on carbohydrates. The fact is no adequate research has ever determined minimum carbohydrate requirements or recommended allowances.

What has complicated the problem is the wide variations in the needs of individuals. Even the same person can exhibit fluctuations from time to time in the metabolic process and change his requirements and needs regarding carbohydrates, fats and proteins.

It has been found recently that overweight persons have a higher tolerance for high fat diets and are less prone to ketonema, similar to acidosis. Overweight persons appear to be able to use up fat for energy at a faster rate and more efficiently.*

Overweight persons are overweight because they do not burn carbohydrate at a normal rate and they store it up as fat instead. A low carbohydrate diet gets results. This we know. But just how is not exactly clear to medical and nutritional authorities.

As to high protein and fat intake and its effect on the body, we have learned much from an excellent research project undertaken in 1928 at the Bellevue Hospital under the direction of Dr. Eugene F. Du Bois who was at that time medical director of the Russell Sage Foundation. Under study controlled conditions—a diet of meat and fat inspired by Eskimo life, yielded no ill effects over the prolonged time of one year. The complete absence of carbohydrate seemed to be a boon. Furthermore, the body derived all of its mineral and vitamin requirements from this all-meat, all-fish, and fat diet. A weight loss and subsequent leveling off at normal weight was noted.

Trouble occurred only when fats were restricted. Fat is a necessary nutrient on a high protein diet. Carbohydrate is apparently not. Because of the close relationship of fat and protein, both as a body requirement and appearance in common foods, the low carbohydrate diet functions very well on "go" and "caution" foods. Where fat must be restricted because of cardiac or other disorder, skip to Chapter VII and follow that diet procedure instead of this one. Gout sufferers might well do likewise. If you have any doubt, consult your physician.

Suffice it to say that the author has had hundreds of cases of obesity respond immediately when carbo-cals have been reduced to the 250 level, without ill effect. In fact, the level of good health has instead risen dramatically. Often people with chronic ailments that do not appear to be related to their overweight condition, see a marked improvement. Ailments that are related to over-

---

* "Nutrition-Endocrine Relationships," Josiah Brown, M. D., Associate Professor of Medicine. University of California at Los Angeles as reported in The Medical Clinics of North America, Vol. 48-No. 5, Sept. 1964.

weight (and there are many) also respond quickly as in the following case:

CASE HISTORY D-101

She Lost Weight On Six Meals A Day

Mrs. L. was a diabetic. At 62 and 185 pounds her health was being critically jeopardized by her weight. She was hungry and thirsty all day. Frequent trips to the refrigerator yielded at least a peanut butter sandwich and usually some fruit and soda for her thirst. She ate rather heftily for a woman and was especially fond of cake, which was bad both for her weight and her diabetic condition.

We sat down and worked out what she would like to eat for breakfast. After selecting several menus to choose from, we moved on to lunch. "Wait a minute," she interjected. "What happened to my mid-morning snack?" No problem. We listed egg salad, veal kidneys, a few more. Then lunch, a 4 P.M. snack, dinner with her husband, and a late night supper—six meals in all. These were then approved by her doctor.

But these were not the meals to which she had been accustomed. They were just as satisfying, and filling, but they were different—they added up to only 300 carbohydrate calories. She enjoyed eating as often and as much as before, but instead of gaining she lost 35 pounds in eight weeks. Her doctor was immensely pleased and found that her need for insulin injections had been lessened. He gave her permission to keep losing until her normal weight of 135 was reached.

Importance of Vitamins and Minerals

It is a foregone conclusion that with your carbo-cals cut to 250 per day, you will lose excess weight and improve your health. Your diet will be balanced. The imbalance brought about in the present carbohydrate century will be corrected. You will be eating right, eating well and enjoying what you are eating.

Aside from the 250 carbo-cal limit, no restrictions have been imposed. You are free to eat what you want and as much as you want. Let's examine this idea of "want." "Want" for food can stem from either emotional or nutritional needs. It is not always easy to tell whether you are bored hungry or hungry hungry. Later, emotional needs, how they cause hunger, and what you can do about it will be discussed. First, let us examine the kind of hunger that stems from actual body need.

The person who is almost always hungry despite the fact that he is eating three square meals a day, and more, may be depriving his body of something it needs. Blood sugar requirements differ so widely with people that it might be in his particular case an extra 50 to 100 carbo-cals is needed over the 250. A physician would be able to confirm this, and would probably advise that the additional carbo-cals be taken in small snacks in between meals to provide the necessary blood sugar level support.

However, chances are it is not a carbohydrate shortage that prompts your body to send up hunger signals. It is much more likely a lack of minerals or vitamins. This is not to say that such a lack commonly causes hunger. It does not. It is more likely to cause broken finger nails and other body deficiencies before it will, if ever, cause hunger. But if hunger is there, and you are eating well, it is a good precaution to supplement your diet with vitamins and mineral additives under the guidance of your physician.

Here are daily dietary allowances recommended by the Food and Nutrition Board of the National Research Council and published by the U. S. Department of Agriculture in their Home and Garden Bulletin No. 72 entitled "Nutritive Value of Foods":

Persons	Calcium (grams)	Iron (mgs.)	Vitamin A (Int. 1 units)	Thiamine (mgs.)	Ribo- Flaven (mgs.)	Niacin (mgs.)	Ascorbic Acid (mgs.)
MEN							
18-35	.8	10	5000	1.2	1.7	19	70
35-55	.8	10	5000	1.0	1.6	17	70
55-75	.8	10	5000	.9	1.3	15	70

Persons	Calcium (grams)	Iron (mgs.)	Vitamin A (Int. 1 units)	Thiamine (mgs.)	Ribo-Flaven (mgs.)	Niacin (mgs.)	Ascorbic Acid (mgs.)
WOMEN							
18-35	.8	15	5000	.8	1.3	14	70
35-55	.8	15	5000	.8	1.2	13	70
55-75	.8	10	5000	.8	1.2	13	70

These are not to be confused with minimum requirements which are generally lower and geared to prevention of deficiency diseases. These are the amounts recommended for a high nutrition level. The units of measurement used are the same usually found on the package of vitamin and other food additives. The quantities in the table are figured for persons at the middle of the age bracket shown, for men 154 pounds and 5 feet 9 inches tall, and for women 128 pounds and 5 feet 4 inches tall. You can make proportionate adjustments up or down in the values if you are off these particular norms.

Food markets in most areas of the country keep a supply of fresh produce available all year around and these recommended allowances are usually far exceeded in the average American's day.

How Much, How Fast

As your well-balanced, suppiemented-with-vitamins-if-necessary eating gets under way, with carbo-cals carefully counted and kept under 250, your weight loss progress chart will begin to reflect results. With some, the line will look like the gentle slope of a meadow. With others, the line will be a precipitous cliff. Still others will have a chart that looks like a staircase.

How fast should weight be lost? A good rule to follow is that 1% of your weight is the maximum you should lose in one week. A 200-pounder should not lose more than two pounds in a week; a 150-pounder, one and one half pounds in a week.

It is better to lose less than this maximum than to exceed it. In case you do exceed it slightly the first week, it may not be necessary to make an adjustment because the first week's loss is often larger than subsequent weeks. However, if your progress chart shows a much greater than 1% loss the first week or averages slightly more than 1% over two or more weeks, add a favorite carbohydrate food once a day to your menu. It might be that a slice of bread or an apple or two will make the difference. Later, you may have to knock it out again to accelerate a lagging loss.

Your proper weight should be what you weighed at 25 if normal at that time. Knowing your proper weight and your present weight you have set a weight loss goal in pounds. Figure what percentage this represents of your present weight and you have just figured how long it will take to get there: If you weigh 150 and your right weight is 120, the 30 pounds you wish to lose is 20% of your present weight. At 1% per week it will take about 20 weeks.

The Crash Program

If your weight loss is too slow, or if it slows up after a few weeks some pounds short of your goal, you may have to curb your appetite to start the progress chart dipping again. But before you give up one mouth watering morsel of lamb shaslik or beef bourguignon, do a fine-tooth comb job on your carbo-cal computations.

Are you counting every course, every item, every portion, where carbo-cals are involved? Are you figuring in every snack and every drink? If you are, and the total is still 250 or under, the only choice left is to cut quantity.

This should be easy. Because if you are overweight, and you are not losing on 250 carbo-cals, you must be eating too blamed much. Whatever the reason for it—assuming it is not a nutritional lack, the time has come to enjoy quality more, and quantity less.

Here are some tips to make the go-easy attitude easier:

Eat slowly, chewing food better and savouring each mouthful.

Put servings on smaller plates; they make portions look bigger.

If you must take seconds, take them in meats and other "go" foods. Avoid seconds in "caution" foods.

If you are a TV muncher, put a bowl of cracked ice on your lap and munch away.

Think thin. Visualize yourself the attractive slender person you will soon be.

Don't be a pig. Help yourself to reasonable portions that you don't have to force yourself to finish.

If you're a refrigerator raider, put "go" food snacks in the way of everything else.

If you need a quick pick-me-up, close your eyes and rest for one minute instead of reaching for a sweet.

If you're eating four or more meals instead of three, try holding off on breakfast until a later hour.

Move salad up so that it is the first course. It will take the edge off your appetite.

If beer is the problem, put yourself on dry wine "spritzers" (wine and soda).

Build up your will power by making affirmative statements out loud about your resolve.

Switch to leaner meats. One ounce of fat contains twice as many total calories as an ounce of lean.

Think of a "caution" food as equaling two portions of a "go" food.

Just for one day, see how little you can eat.

The last suggestion is probably that most important. Eating is a habit. Eating more than you need is a habit. Going one day on the kind of starvation diet that you have been asked in the past to stay on for weeks will break the sequence of your habit, shrink your stomach, and hopefully restore your appetite to more normal levels.

Here is a suggested crash program menu for two days. Pick the one you want. When that day is over, see if you make it two days on the other:

	Day #1	*Day #2*
Breakfast:	Tomato juice	½ cantaloupe
	Two slices Canadian bacon	1 poached egg
	Coffee	Coffee
Lunch:	Cup of clear bouillon	Mixed green salad
	Cottage cheese	Jello
	½ grapefruit	Glass of skimmed milk
	Tea or coffee	
Dinner:	Celery, radish, carrot sticks	Cup of consommé
	Broiled fish	Broiled hamburger steak
	Spinach	Cauliflower
	Melon	½ grapefruit
	Tea or coffee	Tea or coffee

Remember, this is just a two day diet. When you come off it, you can return to your gourmet life of eat all you want. But you will undoubtedly want much less. Continue to practice the previous suggestions as your weight drops.

The progress chart should spell real progress now. The next problem is: can you maintain your weight at the look-on-your-best and feel-your-best level without slipping back to carbohydrate's evil ways. The next chapter tells you how.

6

Eating Well
To . . .

To do you any good, this book must show you the wonderful time of your life. It must lead you along the path of least resistance to food, a path strewn with bones and turkey drumsticks and over which you need never return. Anything less would do you harm, not good. For it would then mean just one more false hope that would send you along a path over which you must return— the two-way path called "diet" which you have taken many times on an unhealthy trip to nowhere.

We all seek an eating way that takes us along a fun-filled tour of the world of food. It is a path in which we step forward with

. . . Maintain Weight

anticipation each day because the previous day was even more of a delight than the day before. Such a path must be free of the need to exert conscious willpower. For there is a limit to how long we can exert this effort; then back we go. To start you on this zestful path, there has had to be a moderate amount of habit-changing. This is always somewhat uncomfortable for a while.

The old tugs at us as we try to depart from it, calls to us as we move away.

If we answer that call, we know the penalty: another off-again on-again poundage cycle with a now-you-see-it, now-you-don't result. All we will have done is to add one more to our list of stop and go diets, and the prophets of doom who criticize the low carbohydrate diet instead of the high carbohydrate dieter will have their day.

You owe it to yourself to enjoy the good life and satisfaction of high protein fun. It will bring you youth, health and happiness. But you also owe it to others to demonstrate, by example, that it can be fun to be thin.

The Food and Drug Administration might well consider the labeling of high carbohydrate foods so that people can be reminded of the damage these foods can do. Meanwhile, the thousands who are flocking to high protein foods are now providing a large-scale demonstration to the public that you can eat well and grow thin.

The previous chapter may have sounded overly attentive to the enemy—carbo-cal. But it had to be in order to get you to be properly wary of this opponent to your health. This switch to proteins is the only change of habit required of you, the only "price" you have to pay to be admitted to the land of Shangri-La with its fountain of youth and perpetually flat stomachs.

Now, with the transition behind you, you can turn to the full enjoyment of your slender self. This chapter will not dwell on the enemy. Instead, it will assume you are dining on baked salmon provencale and duckling "a l'orange" and that you are looking for ways to insure your fun continuing and ever increasing it. So be it.

The Value of Novelty Worn Off

When the canned liquid diet was enjoying its first months of national popularity, some physicians attributed its success at least partly to the novelty of it. Consumer Reports commented that novelties do not long remain novelties. How true.

A high protein diet may be new to you but since it is made up mostly of old friends, it can hardly be called a novelty and that, in a way, is a blessing. A breakfast of Canadian bacon and eggs must soon fit you as comfortably as cornflakes and sugar. There is no reason why you cannot feel just as much at home with a dinner of chopped steak with mushrooms sauteed in butter as you have felt with spaghetti and a hot buttered roll.

The sooner a lusty protein menu fits you like an old shoe the less chance there is that the novelty will wear off and you relapse into sickly sweet ways. Time is on your side. With every passing meal, the gourmet life grows on you, and that white sugary stuff becomes a thing of the past.

Taste is on your side, too. Everyday you are acquiring new taste experiences that you look forward to repeating soon. Sugar and starch become more insipid to your palate.

Well-being is also on your side. "Jim, you look great. Been down to Florida?" . . . "Helen, you seem to look years younger lately. Have you fallen in love?" It is hard to order a banana split at a time like this. You know you owe your new found pep and vitality to an unburdened belly and you're not about to do what the pretty soda fountain sign says. Instead, "No-cal cherry, please." It's good to feel good, and it's good to hear your friends say you look good. You have a lot of things pulling for you. And you've got a good thing going.

During the war when butter became short, the Germans began using a processed animal fat on their bread. Even this became short. With no "ersatz" or substitute in sight, the people learned the trick of placing only a very small amount on their bread, but then placing it upside down in their mouth. In this way the tongue comes into contact with the thin spread and the taste illusion is created of an abundance of spread. When butter returned, the bread promptly did a somersault to its conventional position with the spread on top.

Many diets use taste illusions to cover up for the reduced intake. Celery, carrot sticks, melba toast are all hard and crisp and give the sensation of biting into and chewing a lot of food. When you go back to your regular eating ways, it is a pretty good bet you will zealously avoid celery, carrot sticks and melba toast. Not only are you tired of them, you are tired of being "taken" by the illusion.

High protein dining is free of illusion. It is replete with solid, substantial meals. Find them at Maxim's in Paris or your local diner. Prepare them yourself. This is genuine eating, without duplicity. Enjoyment was never more real. Nothing lurks in your mind to beckon you back to the mainstream; you are in it.

The Pressure of Time

Why did man ever leave this natural, unfattening enjoyment of plenty of high protein food for his carbohydrate treadmill to obesity? The answer lies largely in the time saved by stocking close at hand a variety of farinaceous foods. For early man, grains lent themselves to processing so that they would not spoil. Wheat could be harvested in the summer and fall, ground into flour, and as long as it was kept dry and out of reach of rodents it would last throughout the winter months without fear of getting moldy, rotten or less edible. It was sometimes the only food that he could count on when the winter weather closed in and hunting became difficult.

Later man improved on his methods of refining and preserving grains. He could prepare many varieties of ready-to-eat foods from them that would keep indefinitely, especially in new airtight packages. Sugar, once a luxury, joined these modern foods in cheap abundance. With twentieth century technology, two or three varieties of biscuits in the old time general store burgeoned into hundreds of varieties in the supermarkets. Shelves on Aisle 10 bulge with crackers, wafers, biscuits and cookies. Few women stop to think that bread comes from flour today. It comes from the shelves on Aisle 11: cracked wheat, rye, white, gluten, whole wheat, fortified, French, Italian, and just as many if not more variety of rolls and buns.

For women with more time than others, there is half-baked bread, frozen bread, and ready-to-use rolls. And for a few with lots of time there is even flour to bake bread. Have you tasted any home baked bread lately?

Add to these ready-to-eat grains on Aisles 10 and 11, the cakes and pies on the left side of Aisle 12, the candies on both sides of Aisle 13, the spaghettis, noodles and macaronis on the right side of Aisle 14, the ready-to-eat breakfast cereals on the right side of Aisle 15, and the vast numbers of other ready or partially ready-to-eat processed from grain foods that dot the rest of the store, you begin to realize how far civilized man has come along the carbohydrate way.

But has this trip been necessary? Granted that time is money for some of us, accomplishment for others, is the carbohydrate—that literally turns into body fat as we swallow it—the *only* answer to a breakfast on the run, a sociable cup of coffee, a counter lunch, a quickie snack?

No, it is not. Carbohydrate is an *easy* answer, but man's ingenuity is developing new ways to preserve foodstuffs and now many more types of food can be kept safely for longer and longer periods of time. Are we referring to some new radiation devices or space-age gadgets? They will be along, but meanwhile our refrigeration, freezer, plastic wraps, waxed papers, and metal foils can preserve protein foods as well as the processors have preserved carbohydrate foods.

Preserve protein foods and you preserve your good health. A slice of leftover pot roast is delicious cold. So is a chicken wing. If the roasting pot does not fit in the refrigerator, try taking off the top and covering it with wrap or foil. If it still will not fit, take out the leftover roast and wrap it for cold storage directly or on a plate. All meat and fish leftovers lend themselves to tonight's snack or tomorrow's lunch. And there is nothing more tasty than a cold deviled egg with a dash of paprika. Heating up these leftovers takes time but it is a legitimate option if time is not a factor. If you have no natural gravy left, add a little water to facilitate heating without burning. A teaspoon or two of soy sauce will add fresh zest to the fish.

You can maintain your reduced weight on an even keel by resisting the guiles of the carbohydrate food processors and instead become a protein food preserver yourself.

The Allure of Sugar

Your svelte figure will be under constant attack by sugar. Offered as a reward for good behavior ever since our glands learned how to salivate, we still perform like Pavlov's dogs when sweets are put within reach. We are conditioned to consider chocolates as mouth watering. Rare is the person who does not have to swallow just reading these lines. We react the same to cookies and cakes. Want to make money for your local charity? Hold a cake sale. They always succeed. It would seem we are all hooked.

But it is not just the taste of sugar and sweets that provides the allure. There is also a hunger for sugar, for it is the food that feeds the nerves and the brain. The body can maintain a minimum level of blood sugar even on a starvation diet, but as soon as your blood sugar does drop below normal you feel irritable, depressed and grouchy. That is why diets are so trying. And that is one of the reasons why, when you eat more on a low carbohydrate diet, you feel so much better. With food intake at an adequate level, blood sugar increases and you feel full of drive. This means no craving for sweets and a better disposition.

The so-called Air Force diet, a controlled carbohydrate intake, originated because aircrews were getting fat on their favorite snacks. Doughnuts, soft drinks, candy bars, pies and cakes were being consumed heavily during long hours in flight to provide a high level of energy and relieve boredom. The Air Force, backed by six years of study of controlled carbohydrate diets, circulated its recommendations to crews on how to convert to high protein snacking and eating and leave more of the planes' lifting power for the pay-load.

You can resist the temptation of sweets most successfully by:

1. Eating all you want of high protein "go" foods at every meal, and avoiding self-denial in the interests of dieting. That self-denial boomerangs sooner or later. If the chocolates are passed around, it will be sooner. 2. Realizing that the taste of sweets is an illusion. Everything sweet turns to fat almost as it trickles down your throat. Life is sweet, but life is even sweeter without sweets, and longer.

Sometimes youngsters will have difficulty applying either or both of these defenses, and many of us oldsters, too. More stringent steps may need to be taken to remove the temptation of sweets. Take the case of this young man:

CASE HISTORY C-25

His Family Lowered the Boom On His Weight

Roland, 14, was five feet three, 200 pounds and ill. His pediatrician advised surgery but the surgeon refused to operate. The boy was too fat. His parents and his sister were also overweight but they were trying, and kept themselves in pretty fair check. They thought they had Roland in check, too, but he kept growing, including sideways.

What they did not know was that Roland was stopping at the candy store on his way home from school for lunch. And after lunch he would stop by there again on his way back to school. After school it was the same story. All in all, Roland was sipping and munching away 1200 carbo-cals a day on the outside.

A change or two was suggested. Roland was to eat his lunch in school and his snacks at home. There was always some strawberries and whipped cream waiting for him or a frankfurter to grill if he preferred. He was even given a snack to take to school. The whole family cut down on carbohydrates for breakfast and dinner. Roland was cut back to 250 carbo-cals a day.

The results were immediate: 25 pounds the first month, 15

pounds the second, five the third. He tapered off then. Portions were cut and he continued to lose. At the end of five months he weighed 148 and the combined loss of other members of the family made it an even 100 pounds lost.

Tricks of the Mind

We have the power to undo the conditioning to which we have been subjected through the years, that force which makes us adhere to habits we no longer want, like the sugar habit. The process is called re-conditioning and it can be done through auto-suggestion. When we make a hesitant child taste a new food accompanied by our enthusiastic "oohs" and "aahs" and "isn't it delicious?", we are in effect conditioning the child to enjoy that food. We say he will develop a taste for it; when what we really mean is, we will develop a taste for it for him.

Auto-suggestion can be just as successful as any other types of suggestion. If we tell ourselves over and over again that layer cake tastes like milk of magnesia, the next time a slice is set before us, it most certainly will not taste as good as it did before.

One sure way to put the power of auto-suggestion to work for you is to visualize cakes, pies and sweets as actually turning into fat as you swallow. Tell yourself that they taste like fat even while they are in your mouth. Remind yourself that anything that turns to human fat is bad for you, robbing you of youth and vitality, good looks and attractiveness.

Here are some effective suggestions you can give yourself that will help you to pass up high carbohydrate, potentially lethal, sweets.

> "I know I can be healthier without sweets, so give them up readily."
> "I will maintain my ideal weight, and will not let sweets come between me and this goal".

"I no longer enjoy sweets as I used to do. I understand more
about them, and they are not for me."
"Sugar turns to fat in me. I dislike fat in me or on me."
"I enjoy meat better than sweet. Protein is healthful, sugar is
not."

The way to give these suggestions to yourself effectively is to
speak them aloud and repeat them often. Start the day with an
auto-suggestion session to protect you from the pro-sugar suggestions that will come at you from the newspaper and magazine ads,
radio and television commercials, and grocer's shelves. To come
out even at the end of the day, you really must counteract every
one of these sugary suggestions with an equally powerful anti-
sugar auto-suggestion.

Hypnosis is now being extensively used [1] in assisting people to
make permanent changes in their eating habits, away from carbohydrates and into the realm of gourmet proteins you are now discovering. What hypnosis does, in effect, is to get below the conscious into the sub-conscious where the instruction to like protein
is programmed. All previous conditioning is wiped clean in seconds and new habits automatically substituted.

Teams of specialists have toured the country to conduct clinics
for physicians on the techniques of hypnosis, and many books
have been written on the subject. Self-help through hypnosis is
also possible. Through self-hypnotism you can make your auto-
suggestions much more permanent and effective.* The method
involves attaining a deep state of relaxation, then visualizing your
auto-suggestions.

You can put the power of your mind to work for you by using
your imagination constructively. If you feel like a bite to eat do
not visualize something you know is bad for you. You will suc-
sumb to that visual image as sure as you have a mind. Use your

---

[1] Information may be obtained from *Nassau Institute of Hypnosis*, 21 Bond
Street, Great Neck, N.Y.

* *"How to Reduce and Control Your Weight Through Self-Hypnotism"* by
Sidney Petrie in association with Robert Stone. Prentice-Hall 1965

visioning power to picture steak thumb-bits dripping in gravy or picture cubes of savory gruyere cheese, then succumb to that.

Understand Emotional Pressures

The causes that started us on our high carbohydrate way to begin with are still at work within us despite our new menu and despite the defenses we set up to combat pressures from the world of food around us. These causes are emotional in nature. This does not mean they are not real. They are very real and very powerful. They can set up pressures within us even greater than those from the outside, pressures that can upset the best of new eating patterns.

These emotional factors are highly vulnerable to one tool: understanding. Recognize them and understand them and the most torturing of them can melt away almost instantly never to return.

So it is highly important, if you are to maintain your newly found energy and youth and the high protein ways that made them possible, for you to know a few of the more common reasons why people eat when they are not hungry, or why they eat sweets when they know full well they are committing slow suicide.

When an obese person is upset, he usually heads for the kitchen. This desire to eat at such a time stems from infancy when feeding brought comfort. The infant next feels comfortable even if he has something in his mouth that never reaches his stomach, like his thumb or a pacifier. Through the years eating becomes associated with feeling better. Sometimes cigarettes are chosen to replace the thumb and pacifier, instead of carbohydrates. This is one reason why there are more smokers among the slender.

It is not a conscious thought, like "I'll feel happier if I have something to eat," that prompts the trip to the kitchen. The signal occurs below the level of consciousness in what we call the subconscious. It is the place where compelling forces originate within us. They are forces that cannot be denied. But they are forces that can be turned off by the process of recognizing them when they express themselves, and they are forces that can be re-directed by auto-suggestion.

Typical upset feelings are those that arise when something has gone wrong at the office, when money matters appear discouraging, when you hit another bump on the rocky road called love, when you have an argument, when you are slighted by somebody, when you have feelings of boredom or insecurity.

Next time you step across the kitchen threshold heading for the refrigerator—stop. Are you really hungry? Are you upset about anything? What happened just before you started for the kitchen? Looking back hours later will do no good. Catch yourself at the moment of happening and you can be a successful self-analyst. All it takes is honesty.

Women have been known to overeat because they unconsciously wish to make themselves sexually unattractive. Men have been known to overeat because they unconsciously feel that suicide is the only way out of a business or marital contract. A desire for love, fraternal, parental, etc.—can cause compulsive desires for sweets.

Once you have recognized the emotion that causes the subconscious to ring the dinner bell, you have it partially conquered. It cannot function automatically and irresistably once you have brought it out of the subconscious into the reasoning conscious. In the depths of your subconscious mind it works like a mechanical robot. In the reasoning light of the conscious mind, it can stand only on legs of validity and logic. And how valid or logical can it possibly be to reach into the refrigerator when you are upset!

Suggestion will help to uproot the unwanted motivation, too. If you feel that a particular attitude looks suspiciously like a possible cause of that hungry reach, give yourself positive suggestions to overcome its negative aspects. If it is anger, tell yourself that you are in full control of calm and reason. If it is depression, tell yourself that all that happens is usually for the good even if not recognized as such at the time, and that every day brings new growth.

If it is a crushed ego, tell yourself that you are indestructible and will rise above the situation. If it is tension or frustration, tell yourself that you are relaxed, at ease, happy, and that success is inevitable.

The Two-Pound Danger Signal

Those who take a hard-nosed look at the eat-all-you-want low carbohydrate diet usually admit that you can lose weight eating more calories than on the usual diet. But they add quickly that one seldom eats to excess when on protein and fat, and that actually a big protein day can add up to only 2,000 calories. It is hard to dispute this. Protein foods do satisfy more and there is less chance of a person drifting up to 3,000 calories a day on protein. It is much easier to soar to 3,500 and even 4,000 calories on fast burning, fat producing carbohydrate and not even realize you have been packing it in.

Even if you do hit a 3,000 or more calorie level where more calories are being taken in than expended, the amount of weight gain is far less on protein than on carbohydrate. The body's elimination processes apparently account for the difference.

Your weight is at its best. You want to keep it that way. You are not noticeably eating more, but still the scale has shown a slight increase. (Your progress chart is gone, but you still have your scale). Slight increases come and go. However, consider a two pound increase that comes and does not go as a danger signal. Something is wrong. All else being equal, your total food intake is up above your needs, or carbohydrates have sneaked again through some sweet farinaceous back door.

The longer unwanted pounds stay with you, the harder they seem to be to lose. The faster you act on the two-pound danger signal, the better. The action should be to check carbo-cals first, quantity next. Use all the techniques mentioned in Chapter Five and this chapter to restore your carbohydrate calorie count to near the 250 mark, and to neutralize causes of over-eating.

Chances are the problem can be quickly solved by an impersonal, unprejudiced scrutiny of breakfast, snacks, desserts. Snacks and desserts must bow to "go," "caution" and "stop" signals of your carbohydrate content tables. There are many desserts in the recipe section that will fit nicely into your 250 carbo-cal budget. You will find more snack ideas in Chapter Eight.

The most important correction you may have to make is in your breakfast menu. The U.S. Department of Agriculture in 1949 published the results of a study of breakfasts and their long lasting effect.* After black coffee alone, volunteers became more and more hungry and nervous as the morning wore on. Doughnuts and coffee caused a quick rise in the blood sugar level, but in an hour they caught up with the coffee drinkers in fatigue. Cereals were not much better. The greatest staying power was close to the basic breakfast recommended earlier in this book: orange juice, bacon and eggs, coffee with cream. There was toast, jam and sugar in the coffee added, but this will negate weight loss without greatly affecting the blood sugar level two hours after you have finished breakfast. *The study also showed that the blood sugar level with which you start the day, can set the pace for the rest of the day.* That is why breakfasts deserve your closest attention. They are the most important meal of the day. Proper maintenance of your new figure depends on proper breakfasts.

Adjust Your Muscles

To look your best in your new lines, you should now pay some attention to your body. As you lose weight, muscles that previously became larger to support pounds of fat must now be reduced. Also skin that stretched to accomodate extra volume must now be tightened. You will enjoy doing mild exercises to firm up your figure, prevent wrinkles and sag, and insure a youthful frame.

Remember, these exercises are not weight-reducing in themselves. They are certainly not necessary to do in order to lose weight. Rather are they an important follow-up to your weight

---

* *"The Breakfast Meal in Relation to Blood Sugar Values"*, U.S. Department of Agriculture Circular 827 (1949)

loss as it progresses in order to firm your muscles, restore their tone, increase their strength and flexibility. Your appearance will improve, your carriage will become more erect.

The late President Kennedy created a Council on Physical Fitness. It made recommendations separately for men and for women. These recommendations are clearly spelled out in a program to increase levels of fitness which you can conduct at home without any special equipment. It is called the U.S. Official Physical Fitness Program and can be obtained from the U.S. Superintendent of Documents, Washington 25, D. C.

The program takes only a few minutes a day. It provides several sets of exercises, each set taking you a step further toward a satisfying level of fitness. The exercises are of three general types —warm-up, conditioning and circulatory. They can be done with undue discomfort or fatigue. As you move from level to level, they require increased effort but if your fitness has advanced to a higher level, chances are you will not feel the greater effort you are exerting. A fit person uses less energy for any given movement or effort than a flabby or weak person.

These exercises are singularly appropriate to help men and women along the road to a firm, supple and attractive body. But they are only one of many successful exercise methods. Ask your physician for his recommendations, or check your local library or bookstore for illustrated books on the subject.

Allen Funt, the creator of "Candid Camera," recently lost 40 pounds. It made him feel younger, more vital and energetic. His program took on new life as his enthusiasm caught on among his staff. And he began to exercise regularly to provide his body with the muscular tone it needed in its new life. Exercise made him feel tingly and exuberant.

Moderate exercise deserves a place in your new life too. It need not be calisthenics. It can be golf, tennis, swimming, even dancing. If you once enjoyed a sport but gave it up, losing weight has rolled the years back. Begin again. Have fun keeping fit.

7

The Low Fat,
Low Carbohydrate...

The medical controversy over whether cardiovascular diseases are caused by animal fats has numbers of distinguished authorities defending both sides of the question. The answer may not be known for years. Meanwhile, persons over 40 and those with high blood pressure on advice of physician may want to play it safe pending scientific clarification. This chapter will provide the information on fatty foods needed to convert low carbohydrate menus into low fat, low carbohydrate menus. All others should skip this chapter and go on to Chapter 8 on how to eat out, and in-between meals.

... Diet

At a recent convention of the American Medical Association, three doctors at the vascular research laboratory in a prominent hospital, presented an exhibit purporting to show that man has no business eating meat and that one reason hardening of the arteries is a major killer is that nature intended man to be a vegetarian. These doctors said that their inspection of fossil remains of early man showed that he was herbivorous originally. Following this lead, they fed animal fat to herbivorous rabbits and found that fatty deposits built up in their arteries, while the same diet caused no such reaction in meat-eating animals.

This may be an extreme view, but nevertheless one that has been adopted by an estimated one million vegetarians in this country. Apparently, no survey has been conducted among these vegetarians to determine the incidence, if any, of hardening of the arteries or other cardiovascular irregularities. Such a survey might help to support or deny the contention of the other school of medical opinion which points to the human organism itself as the source of the fatty deposits, rather than the food it consumes. If fatty deposits build up in the arteries of a vegetarian who eats no animal fat, such deposits must be the result of synthesis by his own body.

The author never conducts a weight loss program unless the person consults with his or her physician, and if the person does not have a physician, several are recomended. This is a good moment to remind you that it is always advisable to consult a physician before and during a weight loss program. A physician's decision regarding the proper course for you—fat, or non-fat—may depend on accepted medical theory still in the process of flux and on proclivities of your own body, and its tendency to produce symptoms and danger signals.

The Cholesterol Controversy

In his book, "The Low-Fat Way to Health and Longer Life",* Dr. Lester M. Morrison states: "Atherosclerosis results from an impairment of the body's ability to utilize (or metabolize) normally not only the fats eaten in the diet, but also those that are in the body itself." This seems to tie the two sides of the fat controversy together in a logical way. Dr. Morrison adds that this impairment is further aggravated by the body's inability to withstand stress or tension: and by deficiencies in the supply of

---

* Prentice-Hall, 1958

hormones from vital glands such as the thyroid, adrenals, and sex glands.

Thus it appears that persons subjected to stress or tension must either learn ways to insulate themselves mentally and emotionally from its physical effects or else be wary of high animal fats in their diet. It also appears that persons who have reached the age where glandular activity might be slowing up—and this can come anytime after 40, with hardly anybody immune after 50 to 55—must also be wary of high-fat diets.

This does not mean that everyone who falls into the tension or middle-age brackets needs to avoid high-fat diets. You may fit into both, separately or simultaneously, and still not have to worry because there has been no "impairment of the body's ability to utilize normally" the animal fats and body fats.

The opposite is also true. Not everybody who avoids high-fat diets becomes immune to atherosclerosis. Studies have shown that while about 800 milligrams of cholesterol are in a high-protein, high-fat diet, the normal human liver produces 3,000 milligrams of cholesterol daily. If you continue to consume a high-carbohydrate fare and produce the inevitable body fat, your own fat can cause the same disease. It just becomes an inside job.

On the other side of the fence is Dr. Richard Mackarness of London who authored a book on how to eat fat and grow slim. Dr. Mackarness is of the opinion that it is excess carbohydrates and not calories only that makes a person fat. He declares that a fat man can go on a low calorie diet, but if it is mainly carbohydrate, he will not lose weight; whereas, he will lose weight successfully on a much higher calorie diet if it is mainly protein and fat. What about the harmful effects of fat? Leading authorities feel there is no conclusive scientific support for the suggestion that eating a lot of fat leads to clogging of the arteries. It seems to be much more certain that a loss in weight will benefit than high fat will harm. If a high-fat diet produces that weight loss easier, faster, and more permanently, then it will do more good to use it than to avoid it and suffer the penalties of overweight. A major portion of circulating cholesterol is thought to be synthesized in the liver from carbohydrate and not obtained from the fat we eat at all!

Much of the scientific support claimed for the healthful aspects of low-fat diets is the result of experiments with animals where diets have been imposed that are unnatural to the species. Also in some instances, the metabolic state of the animals has been altered. This makes the direct relevance of such observations to man questionable, unless you believe as the vegetarians do that animal fat is also an unnatural food to man.

Good Fats and Bad Fats

Knowing the whole while that we might be playing a game, and that in reality no fat can do us harm except our own, let us nevertheless examine fats with the same suspicion with which we have examined carbohydrates.

All carbohydrates are the same, but not all fats are said to be the same. Those who point to a correlation of fat to cholesterol content in our arteries level the finger at saturated fats as opposed to unsaturated fats. The saturated fats are the "bad" fats. They raise the cholesterol level in the blood (it is not proven that this high level caused the troublesome arterial deposits). The unsaturated fats are the "good" fats. They can even cause the blood cholesterol level to drop.

What are saturated (bad) fats? What are the unsaturated (good) fats? Saturated fats are animal fats and hydrogenated vegetable fats like margarine and processed cooking fats. They are to be avoided. The unsaturated fats are natural vegetable oils such as corn oil, peanut oil, olive oil, cottonseed oil and the various fish oils and animal oils. Generally speaking, the bad, saturated fats are those which set hard when the pan is left to cool; the good, unsaturated fats, remain fluid when they cool. A more scientific explanation involves describing molecular structure. An unsaturated molecule of fat has room in its structure to add additional fat factors. It is lighter in weight than the saturated fat molecule which is at its maximum weight. It is this weight that causes it to "settle" out of the blood, forming a deposit in the arteries.

Folks who have no reason to suspect coronary and arterial troubles do themselves a disservice in labeling fats "good" and "bad" and should have skipped this chapter according to the instructions at the outset. Even those who do have reason to watch their blood pressure and cholesterol level, should not put a "bad" label on saturated fats or any other food. Permitting the mind to dwell on negative images can "make it so." The immense power of the mind over our body can be exerted in a positive or negative direction. Calling any food bad can actually bring about symptoms that "make it so."

The Chinese tell the story of the man who was invited to tea by his old friend. As they sat in the hut in the light of a kerosene lamp talking about old times, the guest suddenly gulped and grasped his throat. "What is the matter," his host asked. "There was a worm in my tea, and just as I saw it, it entered my mouth and I swallowed it." With that the guest became sick to his stomach. He went to a doctor, but the sickness persisted. Weeks— and several doctors—later the man was at death's door. Then a doctor had an idea. He had the man carried on a stretcher to his friend's house where the incident occurred. He was propped up in the same chair and given a cup of tea. "Look," said the doctor, "See the worm in the cup?" The man nodded feebly. "It is really not a worm, just a reflection from the lamp," the doctor moved the lamp. "See, it has disappeared!" The man straightened visibly in his chair. The doctor repeated the demonstration. Needless to say the man improved steadily and soon regained his health.

The Chinese use the story to illustrate how deadly can be our own thoughts. Let any believable authority call a food "bad" and it will be bad to many of us from then on. Similarly, an innocuous food can be labelled as a health potion and become effectively so to many of us.

The author prefers to bypass the "good" and "bad" labels

placed by many on unsaturated and saturated fats, and instead use the "stop" and "go" technique used on carbohydrates. Saturated fats are "stop" for those who need to be concerned about arterial problems. Unsaturated fats are "go."

How to Avoid Saturated Fats

It is wise to understand the difference between the two kinds of fats, because to try to eliminate all fats not only can cramp your eating style, but will eliminate some vital nutrients your body needs. These essentials are found copiously in the "go" fats, so no nutritional harm can come from completely eliminating the "stop" fats from your diet. Both sides in the cholesterol controversy agree that the "go" fats tend to reduce cholesterol and also reduce weight.

Also both sides agree that it would be better to substitute other protein and fat for the fat you forego rather than to eat that much more sugar and starch. It is not only possible but advisable to stick to your 250 carbo-cal quota, while you shift from "stop" fats to "go" fats.

The saturated or "stop" fats are chiefly the fat on meat and butter fat in cream, milk and butter. (There goes the whipped cream, and many of our cream and butter desserts). Eating lean meat is an easy way of sidestepping the animal fat but even the lean contains a percentage of fat. When physicians take a person off saturated fats they usually try to take him all the way off. There is no quota. Butter is taboo, meats are taboo unless all the fat is cut out or cooked out.

What happens to our gourmet way of life now! Remember the doctor who said to the patient, "Now that we've seen your cardiograph—no drinking, no smoking, no dancing, no sex, no excitement, no golf, no heavy eating—but above all, try to enjoy yourself." Just try. It's a good thing that 90% of the readers have been able to skip this chapter and by this time are deep in restaurant menus or their own refrigerator. For you less fortunate readers, here is the bad news.

Hamburgers are 50% fat—"stop" fat. Breast of lamb is 45%. Even lamb chops are 30%, Leg of lamb drops to 16% and that is the general area of steak (20%), rib roast (18%), and pot roast (11%). The lowest fat content are in the organ meats like sweetbreads and liver, about 5%, but with the exception of liver, they are still high in cholesterol, so you must keep them off the menu.

Poultry and game are around the 5% fat mark, especially the light meat which is several points lower in fat content than the dark meat. Duck and goose are higher, but can be eaten if properly cooked so that the fat has dripped away.

Eggs have 5 grams of fat concentrated in the yolk (and most of it is cholesterol fat). The whites of egg have no fat content. Since egg whites are used in souffles and meringues, keep them in mind as dessert possibilities. Regular milk has about 5% fat. Skimming it cuts the fat as low as 2%. Coffee cream is about 20% and heavy cream is upwards of 35% fat. Cheeses run 25% to 40% fat with the exception of the perennial diet favorite—cottage cheese.

If your eyes are beginning to see the "full life" fade, they fail you not. It is actually impossible to enjoy a gourmet life on a curtailed fat diet. But it is not so restricted a menu that you cannot ask "What's for dinner tonight, dear?" and mean it.

Here are the main changes that you will have to make in your low carbohydrate diet to make it a low-fat diet:

1. Eliminate cream soups. Skim fat from top of other soups.

2. Cut visible fat from all meats before cooking. Cook so that other fat content drains away. Avoid pork, bacon, ham.

3. Avoid organs such as sweetbreads, kidneys, giblets, brains. There is a substance in liver called phospholipids that counteracts the cholesterol content and makes it entirely acceptable.

4. Fish is fine but swing away from salmon, bluefish, herring, mackerel, bass, sardines and caviar.

5. Eliminate milk, butter, cream, egg yolks, and all cheese except the non-creamed cottage cheese.

6. Eliminate salad dressings and gravies that contain fat. Soya oil is fine as are cottonseed, corn and other vegetable oils (except cocoanut).

Considering that there are nearly one thousand foods on our "go" list carbo-cal-wise, the above deletions still leave a great number of building blocks with which to construct a life-time of appetizing menus. See page 214 for a list of major foods and their fat content.

Low-Fat Cookery

Thanks to oft-repeated advice of nutritionists, American housewives are now avoiding many of the cooking habits that have been robbing food of essential nutrients. Vegetables are no longer coming to the table artificially green because soda compounds have been added. Soda destroys vitamins. Nor have they been soaked or cooked in water and the water thrown away, because vitamins dissolve in water. Nor will the truly enlightened housewife peel the vegetables, because the bulk of its minerals then benefit only the garbage pail.

It is especially important to get the fullest nutritional benefit out of every food when on a restricted diet. Raw fruits and vegetables should prevail over cooked, and those that are cooked should not be overcooked. Extremely high temperatures of frying in fat is said to make meat more difficult to digest. Since we are eliminating cooking in fat, the frying process becomes pan broiling with the non-stick pans.

Other methods of cooking meat to minimize fat content are roasting, broiling, braising and stewing. Roasting and broiling should be done at slightly lower temperatures than you are probably now accustomed to. Instead of the usual 350 degrees, roasting at 300 or just slightly over, is recommended. Use racks or broiling pans that permit fat to drain away from the meat. Permit stews to cool, then skim the fat off top, reheat and serve.

Low-Fat Menus

Low-fat, low-carbohydrate breakfasts must replace, bacon, sausage and eggs. Chances are the substitute will be hot or cold cereals, sugar and skim milk. This adds 120 to 150 carbo-cals to breakfast which must come off lunch and dinner in order to stay within the day's quota.

Breakfast undergoes the greatest transformation in switching to restricted fat. Actually broiled fish would be your best bet. No carbohydrates, no fat. But, although it is on the menu at all fine hotels and trans-oceanic steamers, it may be somewhat impractical as daily breakfast food at home, both from the point of view of preparation time, and money.

Roast beef hash or corned beef hash made with a minimum of potatoes, and broiled, rather than fried, is a good breakfast idea. Another is chipped beef in a non-fat cream sauce. Both borrow some carbohydrate in return for the fat. Cottage cheese and fruit make a satisfying breakfast, albeit a change of pace that takes a bit of "getting-to-know-you" orientation. Of course, coffee cream gets watered down to milk, preferably skim, and you will probably want to pep it up with artificial sweetener.

Lunch-time sees little change beyond the meat and cheese variations already mentioned. There are still many salads, cold platters, broiled meat and fish that make up the main course. Gravies must be confined mostly to the *natural juice* varieties. Sauces, now devoid of both fat and flour, derive their basic stock from beef and bouillon cubes and their zest from spices and herbs. Dressings utilize such fat-free constituents as vinegar, egg whites, garlic, tomato puree and catsup, mustard, Worcestershire, tabasco, with vegetable oils getting the green light.

Come dinner time, the low carbohydrate menus survive, with the same exceptions as fatty meats. The same pre-dinner cocktails get a clean bill of health. Bouillons replace cream soups. Desserts become more fluffy as the recipes utilize egg whites but not yolks. So all in all it is not the end of good living. Nor is it exactly the beginning.

Eat All You Can And Lose Weight

New support for the eat-all-you-want-and-still-lose-weight hypothesis has come recently from a European doctor, Dr. Heinz Humplik of Vienna, who has found in 14 years of clinical experience that certain foods require more calories to digest than they supply. This means that the more you eat of these foods, the more weight you lose!

As you might guess, these foods are low in carbohydrates. Most of them are also low in animal fats. They are the very foods with which you will be creating your low-fat, low-carbohydate menus. Dr. Humplik's finding were published in one of the oldest and most respected German medical journals: *Munchener Medizinische Wochenschrift*, Vol. 26: 1183-1186, 1964.

Here is the gist of his findings: A hard-boiled egg requires 92 calories to digest. Since it contains only 80 calories, the body must draw 12 calories from its fat reserve. The more hard-boiled eggs you eat the thinner you get. Perhaps this is not too good an example to select for this chapter since eggs, soft or hard boiled, are high in cholesterol. But the same principle holds for grapefruit, oranges, apples and pears. In the case of the citrus fruits, the pulp must be eaten, too. In the case of the apples and pears, they must not be peeled.

Dr. Humplik lists among the deficit calorie foods lean meats like beef, lamb and chicken, providing they are not fried in bread crumbs; all vegetables except peas, beans, corn and potatoes; all fruits except bananas, seedless grapes, pineapple and melon. He endorses the unsaturated fats in vegetable oils.

Among the fattening foods that provide the body with an excess of calories over what they consume, Dr. Humplik lists fatty meats, some fish, all dairy products such as milk, cream, butter, cheese, all grain and starch products, and sweets.

The findings verify the effectiveness of low-carbohydrate diets, but even more, they provide a theory behind what has heretofore been contention based on experience. A calorie is still a calorie.

But now those who prescribe starvation diets as the only way to lose weight, must re-evaluate their stand. A calorie is not only a calorie, *it is a type of calorie.* There are types of calories that add nothing to the body's daily fuel input. In fact, they use it up. You can actually eat, eat, eat and still lose weight!

A Little Knowledge

Man's sum total of knowledge about his own body's nutritional needs and metabolic processes is still only in its infancy. What makes generalizing so difficult is the fact that people react in different ways to the same foods. It is entirely conceivable, for instance, that although 80 calories in a hard boiled egg is a fixed and determinable figure, the 92 calories expended in its digestion can be variable. Digestion of an egg might require more effort by one body than another, and probably does. One of the reasons may revert back to the fact that even chickens are different. Forgetting the effect of the size of the egg, there are many factors in the life of a chicken that can change the density and nutritional content of an egg, such as the use of electric lights at night to force laying, the nature of the feed, and the pecking opportunities in the yard. Compound this by the differences that derive from the level of human metabolism, state of human health, effect of human attitude and emotion and you have problems with so many variables that even a thoroughly programmed computer could balk.

The very problem of fat and its possible effect on the human artery is complicated rather than clarified by the tomes of clinical evidence to date. Take the effect of cholin, a B vitamin needed to help the body utilize fat. We know it is found abundantly in liver, yeast, rice polish and wheat germ. We know the more fat eaten, the more must be the intake of cholin. But we also know that the amino acid, methionine, is sometimes changed into cholin in the body, and that therefore a deficiency of protein can cause a deficiency of cholin. Then again we also know that betaine, a similar substance found in the same foods and in some others, can take over the work of cholin.

If fat is not being properly utilized by the body, is it because of a diet deficiency of cholin? Or is it a protein deficiency? Or is it a betaine deficiency? Or could there be no real deficiency, but instead a greater need by a particular body that causes a relative deficiency? And if one body does have a greater need than another, what causes this difference?

The answers to the body's peculiarities are the real causes of disease. We treat symptoms today. We sometimes trace cause and effect back a few stages in that treatment. But the basic original cause—like the stock market fluctuations that cause the ulcer, or the tension over a job that cuts off proper digestion—are the factors that man will have to face up to before the medical arts can become an exact science.

When these answers are known, fat restricted diets and no-this-or-that diets may disappear and body malfunctions corrected by counseling and environmental adjustment. And then we might even discover that we can eat more carbohydrate foods without gaining weight!

TABLES OF PERCENTAGES OF FAT IN BASIC FOODS

Following are tables of the extent of fat in basic foods.

FISH

	% Fat
Scallops	0.2
Finnan haddie	0.4
Haddock, smoked	0.4
Pike	0.5
Crab cocktail	1.1
Oysters, canned	1.2
Rock cod	1.3

Clams, raw	1.4
Sturgeon, smoked	1.9
Lobster, broiled	1.9
Crab, canned	2.9
Roe, (Carp or Salmon)	3.0
Mussels	3.3
Halibut	4.0
Sole	5.0
Eels, smoked	6.9
Swordfish	7.1
Codfish, creamed	7.6
Red snapper	9.0
Salmon, smoked	9.3
Salmon, canned	9.6
Anchovies	10.3
Tuna, canned	10.8
Sardines, canned	11.0
Herring, pickled, salted	11.3
Black bass	11.5
Herring, canned	12.4
Abalone	12.5
Perch	12.5
Pickerel	12.5
Shad, broiled	12.6
Caviar, grand sturgeon	15.0
Halibut, smoked	15.0
Caviar, pressed	16.7
Mackeral	18.5
Oysters, fried	20.3

MEATS

% Fat

Beef

Corned beef hash	5.5
Creamed dried beef	9.0
Round steak	11.5

Corned beef	12.0
Round, pot roast	13.0
Club steak	13.0
Sirloin steak	13.0
Rib roast	18.2
Porterhouse steak	20.4
Rump	23.5
Loin roast	28.2
Hamburger	47.4

Lamb Or Mutton

Leg	15.9
Loin chop	25.0
Breast	45.2

Livers

Pork	5.7
Beef	5.8
Calf	5.9

Miscellaneous

Bouillon cubes	2.5
Hash	5.5
Bologna	17.8
Frankfurters	20.8
Pork sausage	27.9
Salami	36.8

Pork

Loin chops	7.2
Loin, roasted	10.0
Rib chops	12.4
Baked ham, smoked	18.5
Boiled ham	20.6
Canadian bacon	33.7
Bacon	55.0

Poultry And Game

Chicken, light meat	4.3
Chicken liver	4.6
Duck	4.7
Turkey, light meat	4.9
Turkey, dark meat	5.3
Chicken, dark meat	6.3
Goose	7.1
Chicken giblets	7.4
Chicken, creamed	19.0

Veal

Loin chop	3.4
Rib chop	3.4
Round, cutlet	4.9
Chuck	5.0

CHEESES

	% Fat
Cottage, skim milk	0.8
Welsh rarebit	8.0
Macaroni and cheese	12.5
Soufflé	24.0
Velveeta	25.0
Liederkranz	25.6
Swiss, processed	26.1
Parmesan	27.4
Pimento, processed	30.5
Brick	30.7
Swiss, European	31.3
Cheddar, American	32.3
Limburger	32.4
Roquefort	33.2
Swiss, American	35.0
Cream, English	36.9
Cream, Philadelphia	43.0
Cream, full	56.0

8

"Eating Out"
And . . .

Eating is the great American pastime; it is always time for a repast. What does the weight-conscious person do about a spontaneous urge for a snack or a spur of the moment "Let's go out for dinner." Deny himself? Refuse? If you are counting calories, yes, because no food is without them. If you are counting carbohydrate calories, there is no need to deprive yourself because, as you now know, there are many foods totally without them.

In Toronto, smokers who want to break the habit can dial for help. By calling a certain number they can listen to a recorded

. . . "In Between" Meals

message in which a convincing voice advises on how to strengthen willpower. Alcoholics Anonymous have a buddy system whenever one can call the other for help if needed. Chances are the first to make available such shoulders to lean on at the right time was Take Off Pounds Sensibly (TOPS). One member often calls another at the moment of temptation. The person on the low-carbohydrate path does not have to set up such will-boosting stations. All he needs is Chapter 8 in this book!

Self-denial is not part of the low carbohydrate way. The urge to "eat out" at restaurants, or in between meals, is always fulfilled. However, it is fulfilled knowledgeably with high protein nutrients that are enjoyable and long lasting. You have found it to be relatively easy to construct such high protein meals from shopping lists. But ordering them from restaurant menus may take a bit more ingenuity and know-how, as may the ability to tread between carbohydrate booby traps at a cocktail party or buffet.

The tantalizing foods that will be served up on the pages that follow are not meant to convince you to throw caution to the winds and enter into a life of "Henry the VIII" abandon. But they are there to be enjoyed. There is a much better chance of your remaining slim through such high protein enjoyment than there is by self-denial.

Look at your weight-watching friends. They launch themselves into a strict diet. They have a slice of burnt toast for breakfast and a bouillon cube for lunch. As an afternoon snack they breathe deeply passing a delicatessen. They can put their whole dinner through the eye of a needle. Do they lose weight? You bet they do. They also very near lose their mind, you as a friend, and certainly their sense of well-being.

Then something else happens. The diet is over. They lost every pound they wanted to and then some. Bravo! Such valor must not go unrewarded. "Let's go to that fancy restaurant and celebrate, dear." Two Manhattans, Vichysoisse, Beef Bourguignon, beer, baked potato, peas, garlic bread, apple pie a la mode, and coffee. It's the beginning of the end. And the end is less than two months away and three pounds or more heavier than at the beginning.

What a price to pay for self-denial! Critics of the low carbohydrate diet would have you believe this is better than the price one pays for self-indulgence. But the choice is not between self-denial and self-indulgence. Rather it is between self-denial and self-control. You can control your weight if you control the kind of calories you consume. Deny yourself calories altogether, and the pendulum must inevitably swing back. Control the character of your calorie intake and you keep things on an even keel.

Living "High On The Hog"

George Bernard Shaw wrote in "Back to Methuselah": *Imagination is the beginning of creation. You imagine what you desire; you will what you imagine, and at last you create what you will.*

There is no doubt that Shaw used this truism in his creative work and that he experienced the imagination-to-creation cycle again and again. Imagination plays an equally vital role in our everyday activities, including eating. Once the imagination roams to the canopied entrance of that charming bistro, you are sure to express your will to go there. And your will is seldom denied. The visit is created. Examine your reaction next time the thought strikes that it's time to check the refrigerator. Your better judgment stays your feet for a minute or two. But then your will prevails, and a snack is created.

The impulse for an in-between snack or a night on the town can stem from basic hunger or more complicated motives far removed from hunger. Some of the many emotional factors that cause the same symptoms as hunger will be covered in the next chapter, but there is one predominant factor that is an outgrowth of our affluent society that deserves a close look here and now. It is the desire to live "high on the hog."

Here imagination runs wild, limited only by bank balances, and even these are circumvented by credit cards, personal loans, and charge accounts. Signs of this affluence are fine clothes, status cars, and being seen in the right places. Then there are the filet mignons, lobsters and pheasants. In a way they gratify even more personally the sense of "having arrived." We deserve our success. There are many ways to rejoice in it, and most of them include good food.

Visualize your desire. The image you see is not that of your-self living "high on the hog" or in any way making a pig or spectacle of yourself. You see yourself enjoying new taste sensa-tions; you hear a cork pop and taste the bouquet of a rare wine; you see a silver casserole cover lifted and smell the aroma of a piquant sauce; you taste a dessert flambé. These are valid images. They create enjoyment.

For some, however, the image is different. And alas, so too is the creation. They are the braggarts and the show-offs. For them, it is more satisfying to tell others they have arrived, than it really is to actually be there. Their image is that of what-so-and-so will say and what so-and-so will think. These are the images of the big self. They create faithfully—down to the 48-inch waist.

On one hand we have the gourmet, the epicure who delights in taste sensations. On the other hand we have the gourmand, the glutton who thinks himself a sensation. And it all starts with the imagining power of the mind.

Obviously, there are two ways to live "high on the hog." One way is to desire new and delicious foods. Pursue this way and you can stay thin. The second way is to desire to be impressive. Pursue this way and you can be a stand-out, a weight stand-out.

None of us like to admit that we eat for any reason other than we are hungry. But the reasons are many. Often they are below the conscious level and we are completely ignorant of them. Others can be discovered by simple-analysis. An honest appraisal of your true motives can lead to some striking discoveries.

Selfish eating might be called the only valid eating. It is eating to please only you. It can seldom lead to gluttonism. Eating is pleasant only when you are hungry. Stuffing oneself beyond normal capacity is distressing, not pleasant. It is a product of mis-use of the imagination.

Proper use of the imagination is your best guarantee that living high will not lead to excesses. Critics have called the high protein, low carbohydrate diet unbalanced and dangerous to the heart, liver and kidneys. Of course, any unbalanced diet is dangerous. But the high protein, low carbohydrate diet becomes unbalanced only when a person is prone to excess. Such a person can make any diet unbalanced, and when permitted to run wild, even among carbohydrates, can endanger not only the heart, liver and kidneys but all other vital organs as well.

Can we control our imagination? Does it take willpower? How is it done? Yes, we can use control. It takes the will to, but little willpower. And it is done by being self-conscious. Get in the habit of observing your thoughts in action, especially when they turn to food. Then, by asking the question—are these thoughts valid? In this way you can expose those images of the mind that have no business being there. The only thoughts that belong are thoughts related to enjoyment of food.

How To Order In a Fine Restaurant

The person who is ignorant of carbohydrate values must resign himself to a weight gain after a meal in a good restaurant. He may go there with every good intention, but these intentions are short-lived. As dinner-time follows the setting sun across our land you can almost hear a million menus open and a million voices mummur, "There goes my diet."

The person who knows carbohydrate values can order in such a way that the meal can be fully enjoyed without falling out of step with weight control. Suppose we unfold a napkin together and examine a typical menu.

Appetizers include broiled mushrooms on toast, chopped chicken liver, pickled herring, prosciutto melon (honeydew with a thin slice of ham), baked clams, shrimp cocktail, tomato juice, pineapple juice. What do you order to keep carbohydrates low?

The answer is, take your pick. The only three items that can affect your carbo-cal budget enough to count is the toast under the mushrooms (the waiter will bring it without toast if you request), the pineapple juice, and the baked clams. It is the bread crumbs mixed in with the minced clams that cause the difficulty, but even so, 20 carbo-cals is about the full extent of the trouble. Clams are fine, and if the menu has Clams Casino or Clams Rockefeller, you are in the clear.

There are many other appetizers offered by restaurants that are right for you. Crabmeat or lobster cocktails often join the more common shrimp cocktail. Melons other than honeydew might be cantaloupe, Cranshaw, or Casaba. All are safely low in carbohydrate. Some restaurants serve a combination of vegetable juices which are all "go." Herring can be replaced by a variety of cold fish fillets including sardines, anchovies, and "fish bits."

What about soups? The soup de jour may be puree mongole (cream of pea combined with cream of tomato) or clam bisque. The standard specialty of the house might be onion soup. Then there may be a choice of cold soups, such as vichysoisse and jelly madrilene. The choice is not as uninhibited as in the appetizers because chances are the cream soups are made with milk not cream and the chef may often use flour to thicken cream soups and bisques. Tomato soup is better than mongole for carbo-cal watchers and mongole is better than pea. Skip the vichysoisse as that is a cream of high-carbohydrate potato, and if you must order New England or Manhattan clam chowder, let the potatoes remain at the bottom of the bowl. Jellied Madrilene is "go"; there probably is not a carbo-cal in a quivering bathtubfull. Onion soup is usually served with a slice of toasted bread already floating in it, and the waiter offers you grated cheese. Too bad it is not the other way around. Accept the cheese, it adds to the flavor, but leave that crusted toast glob of carbohydrates, as it will add nothing but trouble for weight purposes.

The main event is "go" in almost every way. Fish, meat, poultry and game make up entree courses and as you know from your low carbohydrate menu making, all are high protein "go" foods.

The only possible trouble spots are where bread crumbs are used, as in fried chicken or breaded veal cutlets, or where gravy is thickened with flour as may be the case in pot roast, beef bourguignon or some poultry sauces. Avoid meat loaf, meatballs, meat pies, stuffing and hash where bread or potatoes are used as meat fillers, and topping, unless you are prepared to make a place for them in your carbo-cal budget.

Most good restaurants use natural gravies—that is, the juice of the meat itself—stepped up with dry red wine and possibly bouillon cubes. This gravy, even when glamourized with spices and herbs, is "go." Your best bet is to ask the waiter about the type of gravy used. If in doubt, let him serve it with the gravy, then eat around it if it appears starchy.

Skip the bread he puts before you. Better yet, if everybody else at the table is carbohydrate-conscious, ask the waiter not to bring bread. Celery, radishes, and olives are fine to pass the time between courses. So is salad, and you can pick your favorite dressing.

Potatoes, no matter how you escalloppe, gratin or delmonico them, are "whoa!" Choose two vegetables if you are permitted, and make them the non-pulpy ones that you are now featuring on your marketing list.

Desserts present a problem. Naturally the restaurant will roll out its pastry table. If you have eaten heartily and enjoyed your meal, you will have little trouble in passing up this future human cargo for fruit, or cheese and crackers, or jello, etc. Even a small paper cup of biscuit tortoni or fruit ice is high in sugar, higher in sugar than ice cream. Consider the "duck l'orange" that you had for the entree as your enjoyment. Now all you need is something to freshen your taste as you fold up your napkin. There's always grapefruit, melon, or berries and a cup of savory coffee to top off a banquet royal.

Proteins of Other Lands

Part of the fun of eating out is the experiencing of dishes native to other countries. French, Italian, Mexican, Spanish, Chinese and Japanese restaurants abound in most of the large cosmopolitan areas of the United States. In fact, Italian and Chinese restaurants can now be found in almost every small town in most parts of the country.

Folks who visited the 1965 World's Fair had a glimpse of what dining is like around the world. They had a choice of Moroccan couscous, Polynesian chicken, English mutton, Thailand curries, Swedish smorgasbord, Arabian Khomus, Greek shish kebab, Indian tandoori, Lebanese chawavma, Bavarian sauerbraten, Maylasian spiced fish, Jordanese warekinab and scores of other authentic dishes prepared by chefs native to the country. "Go" or "stop"? All "go," except for the side dishes of rice and breads, and the obviously starch-rich items like Belgian waffles. Few countries provide high-carbohydrate main dishes as common items on their daily menus. Ask the waiter about the Polynesian chicken and he will tell you it has been marinated in special sauces. ("No, sir, no bread crumbs or flour.") Ask what chawarma is and you find it is lamb—no carbo-cals. Malaysian spiced fish and bamboo duck as well as their chicken and beef dishes are usually free of ingredients that you need to watch out for, unless you are overly sensitive to hot spices.

The author has dined on pate de foie gras in Paris, venison in London, and Irish Stew in Belfast. The world of food is open to carbohydrate calorie watchers. Only two types of cooking cause problems: One must choose carefully when it comes to Chinese and Italian menus.

Most Cantonese chefs use corn starch liberally in their main dishes as thickening. The popular chow meins and chop sueys are examples of this, compounded by the fact that noodles accompany them. A casserole served as a main course can have as much as 150 carbohydrate content of the vegetables, and the "stop" content of the noodles.

Other Chinese dishes such as Steak har kow, chang chung op (fried duck), egg foo yong (scrape off the gravy), barbecue pork, and butterfly shrimp are more apt to be free of starch. Cantonese lobster is buried in a starchy, pork sauce; but it is buried treasure and worth digging and scraping for. Pass up the rice. As to the fortune cookies, read the fortunes but don't eat the cookies. Mandarin cooking is higher in protein than the Cantonese, if you have a choice of oriental restaurants.

The Italian pasta dominates menus from Florence to Rome. For most Italians it is this dry dough that makes the meal. From the extremely thin vermicelli and capellini d'angelo (angel's hair) to the fat shell forms, there is a veritable world of pasta. All the pastas, especially the varieties of spaghettis, lasagnas and raviolis, too many to list, are all spelled "S-T-O-P." Stay with those redeeming features of the Venetian fare such as veal scallopini, beef Marsala, or shrimp marinara. Italian egg plant is served usually without breading, topped with cheese, and only a minor charge against your carbohydrate account. The antipasto appetizers are a good beginning, but the minestrone soup is a poor if not impossible second course. The anchovy and olive oil salads are budgetable, but skip the spumoni or tortoni ice creams and ask for fruit or cheese instead.

You can eat your way around the world on a high protein, low-carbohydrate itinerary. Exotic souces and rare ingredients may stump you in any accurate carbo-cal counting, but stick to the main protein categories of fish, meat, poultry, eggs, and cheese and a world of food is yours. In Denmark order the Brunkaalssuppe, a brown cabbage soup with just a touch of sweetening. Enjoy the Stegt Suinekam (roast pork) but avoid the Svedsker (prune) stuffing in it.

In Czechoslovakia, the popular Pivni Polevka looks like a harmless cream soup, but it is chock full of beer and sugar, so better try some other soup. Enjoy the Dusene Houby, a delicious sautée of mushrooms, but, if you are interested, the Bramborovenudle are noodles made of potatoes and flour, a team you are anxious to avoid confronting.

Finland's Etikkasilkat (pickled herring) is marinated in a sauce that includes sugar, but not enough arrives with the delicious smorgasbords to worry about. There will be only about a teaspoon of flour in your cup of Kurkkukeitto (cucumber soup), very well worth in taste the cost of 10 to 15 carbo-cals.

The middle east and orient throw rice in your protein way at every gustatory step, but the tourist can well afford the many other choices out of reach of their people but available in their restaurants. Certainly the blessing of high protein dining is apparent to the traveler, whose exciting culinary fare yields him his money's worth in plane and boat fare at constant weight, while the average calorie-counting dieter must miss this flavor of travel or else arrive home with unwanted, excess personal baggage.

Eating Between Meals

The literature on diets can fill a library. Much of it is completely bewildering because of conflicting facts and assertions. Some of the literature, put out by private interests, carries the arguments for weight control methods to extremes. To bring some order out of chaos, there is a growing feeling among Washington legislators that a study of diets be made by a panel of medical and nutritional experts to ascertain complex interrelationships between diets and body health, and the effects of reducing remedies. If started, it would certainly be a worthwhile project, providing it would be vast enough in scope to cover the many different ways people can react to identical diets.

One of the controversies that might be resolved is the effect of eating between meals. Opinion is varied: There is a candy booklet that suggests that if you eat candy between meals, you spoil your appetite and therefore eat less and there is the "six snack-no meal" diet that eliminates the usual three meals a day altogether and substitutes six elegant between-meal type snacks in their place.

Even within the ranks of proponents of low-carbohydrate diets, there are those who believe that the high protein breakfasts, lunches and dinners inhibit the desire for snacks because of their greater satiating power; and others who feel that the urge for snacks is increased because of the bodies' need for quick (carbohydrate) energy.

Which is true? Will you be starting to fade at 10 A.M. or just gathering momentum. Will you need a late afternoon pick-me-up or will you still be going "gung-ho" at 5 P.M. The author's experience over the years with thousands of cases points to both sides being right. The low-carbohydrate diet is not likely to change the day-to-day habits of the individual. If you are in the habit of a couple of quick ones in the late afternoon, substituting a chopped sirloin steak for a hamburger is not going to change any-thing except your weight. If you are in the habit of cold cereal breakfasts and of quitting the drawing board for a ten minute break over a cup of java, your bacon and eggs breakfast is not likely to change that.

What may have to be changed is the danish that goes with the coffee and the kind of cocktail that goes with the hour. Morning or afternoon coffee breaks present a challenge to our low-carbo-hydrate way of life. It is so easy to say toasted English, or cruller, or jelly doughnut, or prune danish. Coffee all by itself is unthinkable, as unfinished as a pucker without a kiss. What high protein, quickly servable foods are there? And can you get them at the usual counter or mobile coffee break unit? The answer is there are many, yes; but no, they are not likely to be available even at large coffee shop counters or the most well equipped coffee vendors. Certainly not in this decade will they be carrying fresh fruit, melon or berries; or even cheese slices or soy bean wafers.

The in-between coffee drinker must solve his or her problem in his or her own way. Working man or student, working girl or housewife, your ingenuity must be brought into play with your own personal taste the judge. An important factor will be whether you are on a weight-loss or weight-maintenance program. If it is weight-loss, you may have to pucker without that kiss—coffee alone. If you have leveled off, there may be a way to fit half of a toasted English (with plenty of butter) into your carbohydrate budget.

At home, the coffee break, afternoon bite, and midnight snack are solved more easily. All it takes is a little planning. The fruit can be unfrozen the night before, or chilled as the case might be. Leftovers can become less a matter of today's chance and more a matter of yesterday's pre-meditated extravagance. How nice to find a cold chicken leg or wing with the flavor carefully wrapped in. Or the carcass of a duck to explore. Or a nearly bared roast leg of lamb to pick away at. Remember the livers you did not serve with the chicken? They will take but two minutes on the range. Try new cheeses. Sautée some mushrooms. Keep some hard boiled eggs ready to peel. Open a can of Swedish meatballs, smoked oysters, or minced clams.

What To Eat or Drink at Parties

If you head for the bar at the end of the working day, then whiskey, vodka, rum, gin, brandy or dry wines are your best bet. This applies to the cocktail party, of course, as well. There are two good reasons for ordering your drinks straight, instead of mixed.

1. Chances are the mixing ingredients are carbohydrate-heavy, like carbonated mixes and sugar.

2. A straight shot is one ounce, but a cocktail is two to three ounces. Martinis are not made with sugar and contain no carbohydrate when dry, just a trace from extra dry Vermouth. Use French Vermouth as it is much lower in carbohydrate than Italian. Avoid beer, sweet wine, and cordials. Don't reach for the peanuts or potato chips. If the bar puts out cheese, cut yourself some cubes or slices that you can eat conveniently without a cracker. At home, keep a supply of roasted pumpkin seeds or fried bacon rind, found at most supermarkets.

If Pekoe or Oolong is your cup of tea, and an afternoon tea party your weakness—or strength—your only problem is what to serve on that platter in the center of the table. Cake and cookies have carved out a traditional niche for themselves at a tea break, so any substitute must of necessity be sort of shattering. But growth and maturity in life is said to be the casting off of old patterns for new, and if this particular pattern is not "chucked out," the growth will most surely be in the body—where it is not wanted.

What can take the cake's place? One idea—open sandwiches. No, this is not a typographical error. You can enjoy open sandwiches providing you are willing to adapt them to your protein way. This can be done by means of the low-carbohydrate soybean cracker, or you can borrow an idea from Polynesia and the Far East and serve your salmon salad or tuna spread on crisp lettuce leaves. Strawberries and whipped cream are always welcome at an afternoon tea. But you take it from here. There are many possibilities, albeit all novel; the only limits are your ingenuity, taste, and carbohydrate budget.

You may want to substitute a champagne punch for the tea. This brings you a step closer to the cocktail party, takes you away from obligation to sweets, and opens up a whole vista of cocktail party hors d'oeuvres. A favorite recipe for champagne punch calls for one bottle of domestic sauterne for each bottle of dry champagne. Add a few jiggers of brandy and the juice from a lemon and an orange.

At a cocktail party, martinis are your favorite mixed drink, champagne flows freely, and the tinkle of ice sings a ballad of scotch, bourbon or rye on the rocks. That hot tray making the rounds has an army of little party toothpicks each with a tiny captured frankfurt or a miniature meatball. Another tray has a separate color toothpick for each kind of cheese tidbit. The gourmets need not see the color chart; they can identify each cheese by name. How about your guests?

Those are fish bits on the platter over there; three types of herring, an anchovy, and two types of sardines. The crowd at the end of the table is grouped around the shrimp, which has a spicy cocktail sauce. Next to it is the black and red caviar ringed with soy bean crackers. The crackers are also supplied next to that onion dip. Another sauce of mayonnaise and sour cream is ringed by small pieces of raw cauliflower that spur words of praise for the hostess' originality.

Party Fun Without Gain

The festivity of a party can be captured in a high protein atmosphere, perhaps even more genuinely than when carbohydrates have been invited. The blankets around the little pigs (franks) are in reality wet blankets, that leave you a little heavier and less able to enjoy the next party and living in-between. The bread that carries a spread is a sad sack indeed. The sweets are out of place and can add to you in the wrong places.

A recent survey of 7,000 persons by the U. S. Public Health Service reveals women to measure a bit more across the beam than men. The measurements were taken in a seated position using a light but sure contact to compress the clothing. From port to starboard it was 14 inches for the men, 14.4 inches for the women. Somehow men have known this fact all the while, despite girdles and all. And they have liked it. Women today seem to be overly conscious of what they think is padding—but what is in reality their feminine endowment.

It is unhealthy to be overweight. But it is not healthy to be obsessed with a desire to be as straight as the size 8, or size 10 models that stare macabre-like from the pages of fashion magazines, even if you make your living as a model. In this age of tension and anxiety, the relaxation that comes at a party or social get-together of two or twenty is far more therapeutic and health-producing than would be your building a wall of abstention between yourself and the fun because of a few calories.

Calories count. But so does the rapid-fire conversation, the witty interplay, the laughs. And they may burn off more calories than abstention can prevent. Deprive yourself of the kind of diversion and relaxation from every-day problems that parties produce and you may be building up the very condition that brings on overeating in the first place. Partying is a constant whirl in many urban and suburban circles, but on the average it is underdone by our present society. The result is loneliness and boredom that lead to private parties between us and the refrigerator. Parties without fun; eating and drinking without hunger or thirst.

Diets come and go. The only one that seems to have arrived with a one-way ticket is the low carbohydrate diet, and maybe it is not really a diet but a return to natural, balanced eating.

This is based on a very simple fact, but from that fact come several important derivatives. That fact is: carbohydrate calories put weight on you easier than do protein or fat calories. Because of this:

1. You can eat more in protein calories and still lose weight.

2. The protein foods you replace carbohydrates with give more lasting satisfaction.

3. Judiciously selected, 250 carbohydrate calories per day provide a generous choice of nourishing foods.

4. Hunger and deprivation are no longer necessary in order to lose weight.

5. Family and social eating habits do not have to be eliminated or cut back, but only revised.

6. Willpower is needed only to make these revisions, not to make sacrifices.

7. These revisions then become habits, eliminating the need for willpower entirely.

8. With exertion of willpower eliminated, there can be no relapse because of weakened willpower.

9. Without relapse, weight loss is permanent.

It is logical to attack the plan by saying that carbohydrates in check leave protein or fat that can be consumed in excess. Therefore, there is a chance that the low-carbohydrate diet can be high in certain fats considered by some authorities to be dangerous for some people. Granted. But shall we write off this infallible, health-producing method because it can be abused? It is like saying we must ban aspirin because someone may hurt themselves by taking an overdose.

The more you can enjoy your low carbohydrate eating fun, the better the chance that you will adopt it as a permanent way of life. In so doing, you are choosing a slimmer figure, bidding adieu to up-and down weight cycles, and adding youth and years to your life.

9

Understanding
Your . . .

Some people can eat anything and everything and stay thin. Others seem to gain weight no matter how careful they seem to be. Both types of people have active appetites. But those who gain weight must have appetites that do not register hunger accurately. Their furnace is not burning as furiously as a thin person's, yet it keeps calling for as much fuel.

Appetite is the desire for food. Hunger is the need for food. If appetite and hunger were in step with each other, fifty million weight watchers in this country could relax their vigil. But they are not in step, and it is usually appetite's fault.

. . . Appetite

Appetite can ring the dinner bell, just as you have folded your napkin after a big meal. It can sound the alarm in the middle of the night or at a crucial moment in an important transaction. It has even been known to keep ringing with no eating way to turn it off.

Masked as hunger, appetite is not recognizable. We are hungry and can have hunger pains. We never say we suffer from appetite. If we acknowledge that we have an appetite, we say it is because we are hungry.

If we could unmask "hunger" and find it is really appetite masquerading as hunger, would we be better able to deny its unrelenting insistence that we eat? The answer is "yes, but." Yes— if you could understand just what emotional factors were touching off your appetite, you may be less likely to succumb to it. But—these factors may be so deeply buried in the personality that only lengthy psycho-analysis could bring them to light.

It cannot hurt anyone to understand how the urge to eat comes about, and it certainly may lead to a more wholesome attitude towards eating. This understanding is far more valid an approach than attempting to stifle the appetite with chemical depressants. This use of pills is somewhat like trying to stop a baby from crying by putting your hand over its mouth. Take the pills away and appetite resumes more bearingly than before. Keep them in use for too long a time and they can be lethal. Appetite fools most people most of the time. Once understood, it can fool less people, less often.

The Appestat

When you think of the number of people that are writing their own epitaphs: "Death came prematurely from obesity," you would think that a great deal of information about the appetite would be available to physicians and laymen. Actually, very little has been printed on this subject, compared to what has been printed on the general subject of being overweight.

Appetite is a mechanism that operates as other automatic body arrangements which bring about the results desired by influencing behavior. An itch encourages us to scratch. A throat tickle impels a cough. Appetite demands satisfaction from food.

Just as an itch can come from something as non-functional as watching someone else scratch or the throat tickle from a cigarette, so can appetite call for eating when eating is not really called for. But it is pretty hard, if not impossible, to deny that scratch or suppress that cough even if we understand how or why the signals are getting crossed.

A thermostat that is located where a cold draft from the front door hits it can send the furnace urgent signals for more heat even though the house is warm. The appetite, sometimes called the appestat because it automatically signals for more fuel for the body, can also misfunction for a number of reasons which will be discussed in this chapter.

Even persons who can normally tell the difference between their appetite and their hunger can be taken in, as when some emotional crisis occurs and the subconscious decides that oral satisfaction is wanted and the only way it is going to get it is if "genuine" hunger pains are sent up. It behooves us to recognize not only the difference between appetite as signaling for the pleasure of eating, and hunger as signaling for the need to eat, but also to be alert for the time when appetite dresses in hunger's clothing. Just as a father-to-be can suffer sympathetic labor pains that are very real, so can expectant mouths induce stomach pangs that are often indistinguishable from hunger pains. The same logic that reassures the father is usually just as effective: "I just ate. It is impossible for me to be hungry. It must be something else. What can that something else be?"

Dr. Norman Jolliffe was credited with coining the word "appestat." He located it in the hypothalamus, which is near the pituitary gland at the base of the brain. He claimed that when this area of the brain was damaged in rats, they ate like gluttons and soon weighed twice as much as normal rats. However, later experiments with the thalamus failed to produce similar obesity in other types of mammals.

Perhaps the appestat can be located some day, and then even physically adjusted. But meanwhile it can be adjusted only by untraining and retraining, and by emotional changes.

Retrain The Appestat

One way that this can be done is illustrated by this case history:

CASE HISTORY 1-41

Mrs. Ruth K., 38, was the wife of a lawyer. She weighed 172 pounds when I put her on the scale the first time she came to the office. One reason for her overweight was that she was always hungry at night. She woke up consistently in the early morning hours, went to the icebox, and made herself a sandwich or ate a piece of cake.

Obviously this was a case of an appestat reacting to some emotional need rather than bodily need. But to her, it was identically the same as hunger and it had to be satisfied.

First, I had her prepare somewhat different snacks with less carbo-cal content, before she went to bed. When she made her 3 A.M. foray to the refrigerator she found orange slices, melon, fresh fruit salad awaiting her. Sometimes she prepared rolled up lettuce leaves with tuna salad inside. We stayed away from heavier items, such as steak slices or cheese, because this was not just an operation to lower carbohydrate intake, it was also a retraining of the appestat. Similar reductions in carbo-cal were made in her other meals and within a month she lost 18 pounds.

The next step in this retraining of the appestat was removing the need for her to get out of bed to have her post-midnight snack. The fruit was placed on a table at her bedside. She awoke as usual, had a few bites, went back to sleep. Her psychological need to wake up, for whatever deeply hidden cause, was still satisfied.

Two oranges were then all that were placed by the bed. They were never finished, and occasionally never touched. Soon she was sleeping through the night, secure in the fact that the food was by her side if she "needed" it. Naturally, with one unwanted meal eliminated, her weight loss continued at a happy rate.

There is no known psychological problem that requires apple pie to cure it. The food that it drives one to eat is a substitute for the satisfaction that the problem demands. However, if food is taken away as a substitute, some other substitute will be sought by the subconscious. It may turn out to be an appetite for sex, for cigarettes, for chewing gum; or a sudden interest in new hobbies, in television, or in card games. It may even be expressed more naturally in a new verve and enthusiasm in business, home or social affairs.

When, as in the instance of the above case history, protein is substituted for carbohydrates, no other substitute is needed. Food continues to be the crutch. This is always a good first step, because it gets rid of unwanted carbo-cals while maintaining a permissive attitude, free of hostility and its often drastic counter-effects.

The second step is the gradual diminution of the effects. This permits a gradual adoption of a substitute, enhancing the probability that it will be along a path of little social resistance. A sudden need of a substitute can carry with it a high emotional voltage that can jump wide gaps in behavior patterns. By placing the snack progressively closer and easier to get at from the bed, Mrs. K. made a gradual transition to new attitudes. There was no need to know what they were, just as there was no need for lengthy psycho-analysis to get at the original cause.

From the author's experience with hundreds of analogous cases, there emerges this successful two-step procedure for untraining or retraining the appetite where special unwanted habits are present:

Step One: - Translate the habit into its low-carbohydrate counterpart by merely substituting one food for another.

Step Two: - Gradually diminish the unwanted effects of the habit in progressive stages over a comfortable period of time.

Frontal Assault on Over-Eating

There may be no special unwanted eating habits to cope with, just the habit of eating too much. Retraining the appestat in its overall operation requires the same kind of repetitive practice as improving a golf swing or learning a new piece of music on the piano. It means putting yourself through those paces that you want to become a natural habit, again and again.

Six lessons may correct a golf swing, six hours may permit mastery at the piano, but chances are it will take all of six weeks to untrain and retrain your appestat. Persons who go on the usual low-calorie semi-starvation diet undergo this retraining, but it is usually not quite complete—for two reasons—so the appestat resumes its weight-adding behavior as soon as the diet ends. Those two reasons are: 1. The time is insufficient for retraining, 2. The procedure is acknowledged to be temporary and therefore not a retraining. To properly retrain the appestat we must:

1. Recognize what constitutes over-eating.
2. Restore quantities to normal levels and keep them there for six weeks or more.
3. Re-balance the diet by substituting long lasting proteins for short-lived carbohydrates.
4. Reaffirm weight control goals.
5. Review personality traits that could be affecting the appetite.
6. Revise causative mental attitudes in a positive and wholesome direction.

These may look like six simple steps, but they require effort, discipline and perseverance. The best part of the whole procedure is that it is a short story with a happy ending. If you read this six months ago and went through a retraining of your appetite, you could not only be 30 or 40 pounds lighter by now but could have arrived at your right weight weeks ago, and could have forgotten all about the retraining period by this time. What is more, you would know that the days of diets were over, that you were permanently slim, and that you were now one of those fortunate persons who could eat all they wanted and not give it a thought.

The low-carbohydrate way of eating provides a sure-fire method of weight loss without under-eating as most other diets require. However, it will not provide the same weight loss to over-eaters. Over-eaters need not retrain their appetite by under-eating, but they must practice three-square-meal living for a while. When they emerge from that period, they are not likely to return to over-eating.

Anything above three square meals a day is over-eating. Anything above an occasional second portion is likely to be evidence of over-eating. Anything above an occasional coffee break or midnight snack is also evidence of over-eating. Use the menu on page 61 as a guide to normal eating volume. If it looks skimpy to you, you had better plan to enroll right now in the "School of Normal Eating" and accept an education concerning the faults of your past dietary practice. Once you realize you are over-eating, it is easier to seek the cause. Mortality figures are meaningless when food is in front of you. A mirror is better.

Use the low-carbohydrate way of eating to restore normal quantity. It will help you to get along on less quantity because of the way proteins keep you satisfied for longer periods. Use the list of suggestions on page 186 to cut down on over-eating. Enjoy interesting foods and a diversity of preparation ways, as increased interest and diversity can more than make up for reductions in sheer quantity.

Personality Traits That Affect Appetite

When a person is faced by a situation he cannot understand or with which he cannot cope, a state of anxiety usually develops. It is this anxiety, whether we are conscious of it or not, that can produce the personality traits for which over-eating can be a symptom. It is better to be conscious of these anxieties than not, because the chances are then better that they can be resolved. But even if you are conscious of them, the sub-conscious can persist in manifesting the symptoms and may even obstruct your attempts to correct them.

The intolerable situations in life that can cause obesity via anxiety are countless. Examine a thousand cases and every one will be different, but certain basic emotions or attitudes dominate all of them and provide a way to classify them. It is not intended that the reader recognize himself or herself in any of the situations that follow, rather it is hoped that these situations illustrate the way anxiety can build up. Keep in mind that there is a resistance by the conscious mind to recognizing one's own anxieties, but keep in mind also that six weeks of conscientious appetite retraining may be for nought unless a sincere effort at objective self-examination is made.

The spectrum of anxiety runs from fear of sex on the part of young people to fear of being without it on the part of older people; from insecurity on the part of some to boredom in others; from resentment and hostility to aggression and guilt.

A frustrated ability to express oneself is often compensated for by eating. The man who must do things the way his boss wants them done is ripe. So is the child for which mother does everything. Or the mother whose housework and baby-sitting now keeps her from enjoying the exciting activities of the business world.

The sexual relationship springs from a similar procreative drive. Social taboos may consciously inhibit the sexual drive but the subconscious must find some other outlet for its frustration and the kitchen refrigerator oftimes plays the role of secret lover. It is no secret to the analyst but to the one who is involved it can remain an unbreakable habit until there is a resolution of the sex problem.

Insecurity about the future can arise in many ways. Most common is the financial insecurity that is the lot of most people on earth. But there is also insecurity about a job which can stem more from imagined than real factors. There is insecurity in love where the mind can dwell on the infidelities of the spouse, also usually more often imagined than real.

Can you imagine the results of low calorie starvation diets on people inwardly wrestling with any of these problems? It takes the floor right out from under them. They are as smokers without a cigarette in sight; alcoholics in a dry State; a tightrope walker without a balancing stick. Little wonder that they cheat, then innocently deny it at their weekly visit to their doctor when the scale registers "no loss." It is easier to face the music than the empty despair.

The low carbohydrate diet is not a starvation diet. So it brings with it no such emotional shock. If food is your security, you remain secure. If food is your relief from boredom, you are not bored. Whatever the reason for food to be used as a crutch, the crutch remains to be leaned on until that reason can be ferreted out, understood, and eventually dissolved in the maturing personality. Meanwhile, weight can be controlled and weight gain prevented. If appetite can also be controlled, weight loss can occur even before the emotional cause is alleviated.

This becomes very important where a bright lift to a drooping morale is all that is needed to turn the tables on a problem. That lift can come from pounds lost. A better physique, a more attractive figure, and increased energy can dissipate the very emotional doldrums that brought about the excess poundage to begin with. But trying to attain these on a starvation diet is like trying to drive forward in reverse gear.

The writer could offer case history after case history in which emotional conflicts lead to all types of overeating from aggressive devouring impulses to simple needs for oral stimulation; not one would be a situation of value to the reader by analogy or similarity, because every person is unique and his or her problems are unique.

How To Probe The Subconscious for Appetite Secrets

Hidden causes for an overactive appestat need not remain in the hidden subconscious forever. Nor do their discovery necessarily require psychiatric assistance. Every day we draw on the subconscious for answers. We might just as well put in our order for this vital one.

There are several methods that are effective in inducing the subconscious to divulge hidden causes of our actions or feelings. Everybody has experienced at one time or another the frustration of a name or place that cannot be remembered. "It's right on the tip of my tongue," we say. What we really mean is that it is right on the edge of our conscious mind. And chances are that is where it remains until we stop trying. Some time later, when we have forgotten the dilemma, the information arrives. All the methods for probing the subconscious requires this same non-interference by the conscious. When you stop trying, the answer comes. But first you must call for it.

In the case of remembering a name or place, you literally asked yourself for the answer. Suppose you asked yourself for the answer to this question: "Why do I eat too much or too often?" The answer will not be on the tip of your tongue. But if you forget that you asked for it, the answer will come. It may not come for an hour, a day or a week. However, you will get an apparently uninvited thought regarding that problem. You may remember the day your baby sister was born. (Why is that memory popping into my mind? Could I have been jealous and felt I was not loved by my parents? How silly!)

Those two words "How Silly" can well mean the end of over-eating. For when a cause that is no longer valid is fished out of the subconscious and evaluated by the conscious, its power over you is gone.

You can increase your chances of getting an answer from the subconscious by asking for it more effectively. The more you want the answer, the more emotion-packed is your request. A listless request will fail. An intense request, even bordering on prayer, is more likely to succeed.

There is a way to talk to the subconscious more directly. Relaxation has a way of folding aside the conscious mind and exposing the subconscious. If you can relax deeply and keep your mind as close to blank as you can, then when you ask for the answer to a problem, you will be amazed how fast and vividly you can get the answer.

If you find it difficult to approach your subconscious for assistance, you can use a conscious deductive method to ferret out emotional causes for over-eating. Use the system outlined in Chapter 2 to record all of your food intake for a period of days.

But instead of just listing the foods and portions, write down a brief record of what happened just before you ate and what your feelings and state of morale were at the time.

Analysis by you may reveal an emotion-food relationship— coffee breaks after personality clashes, or money worries, or thinking of someone; second and third portions after an especially hard day at the office; or an especially aggravating time with the kids.

Write down everything that you can think of even though it does not seem pertinent at the time. You may feel you have the best mother-in-law in the world, but if she appears in your notes frequently and in close time proximity to your food forays, it is a good bet that you and the old girl have had some problem that was never quite faced.

Old Problems Versus New

An old problem, long since solved, can continue to do its fattening work as if it still is a current issue. Something that happened to you as a child can still trigger "hunger" though long since forgotten and totally meaningless today. Pull it out of the depths of the mind into the cold white light of logical scrutiny and the obvious unrelatedness to your life today makes you reject it as of any importance. It was vitally important when it happened and it entered your memory storehouse with that "vitally important" label. Today, as you experience it again through self-analysis, the event is returned to your memory storehouse with a new label, "reject." From that moment on it is eliminated as a subconscious force that can produce false hunger and create abnormal appetites.

On the other hand, if the problem is current, the mere recognition of it does very little to remove the symptom: over-eating. Putting a persistent attitude or emotion under that same cold white light of logical scrutiny can be painful, if that problem is a current one which, rather than face, you have been burying in an avalanche of indigestion.

It is easier to eat to forget than not eat and face, so easy that we do it automatically without thinking. That is why it can come as a surprise that we are doing this at all. Once we know, we may be reminded of it at every turn of the fork, but most of us will not put the fork down, that is, until the problem is solved.

Easier said than done, you say. Right. Solutions are not easy to come by. But one thing is sure, if a problem is known to exist, it is a step closer to its end. If, in addition, the problem is thoroughly identified, it is another step closer to finis. And, finally, if the identified problem is known to be causing another and possibly more serious problem—obesity—the stage is set for apathy to bow to a vigorous attack.

Emotional factors, whether stemming from yesterday's or today's problems, must be neutralized if chicken luau is to be savoured by a gourmet appetite, rather than wolfed down to fill a void, and champagne sipped for its vintage, not gulped by an unquenchable thirst.

Bypasses Are Dead Ends

If you are eating too much, you have an eating problem that is a matter of life and death. It is worth many hours of soul-searching to identify the cause, though it be trivia from the past. Should that cause reside in a present environmental situation, all the more reason to expend effort to resolve it.

There is no way to side-step the issue permanently. Millions try it every year and fail. They turn to food diets, steam baths, and purgatives. They hike, pedal and run; submit to the poundings of masseurs; and rock and roll on vibration tables and couches. The pounds come off. The goal is reached. The pounds return.

Little wonder that internists and general practitioners often have little patience with their "big" patients. They must turn treats into treatments and then watch human frailty succumb to the irresistible force of food. This frailty has paved the way for the use of the so-called obesity specialist who substitutes pills for discipline.

Frowned on by the medical profession, but engaged in by some of its members, the obesity specialist dispenses pills and capsules in assembly-line fashion, usually after only superficial examination.

The pills often include such dangerous and powerful substances as thyroid extract and digitalis. Some use appetite depressants and de-hydrating drugs, phenobarbital and amphetamines, laxatives and vitamins.

Thus are the glands and nervous system subjected to false stimulants and tranquilizers and the over-weight person literally shrunk to proper size. But the day of reckoning is always close at hand. Once the treatment ceases, the appestat returns to normal abnormality and the status to obese quo.

Similarly, diets are effective only when they are not used to by-pass the cause of overweight but rather to restore proper weight after the cause has been corrected. Used otherwise a diet is a dead-end street over which weight must return to where it started from.

That is why fifty million calorie-conscious Americans find dieting a frustrating roller coaster with every weekend a jolt, every season a dip or a rise, and every circuitous ride a discouraging repeat.

Respect Your True Appetite

Rid of intruders, the genuine appetite is a blessing. Free of erroneous conditioning, its behaviour is to be respected, its urgings obeyed without guilt or conscience pangs.

Literature is replete with tales of voracious appetites, like the baron that consumed a whole leg of mutton, a large capon, and a quarter of a large cheese, all washed down by a bottle of wine. Or take King Henry VIII himself. For some reason appetite in those days was considered to increase in direct proportion to the dignity of the personage. Perhaps it had something to do with that dignity having been inherited rather than earned. But whatever, it did not have a genuine ring.

True appetite is the clarion call of life itself. Plants and animals renew themselves through the intake of tissue building material. Energy for sustenance is provided by nourishing food. Appetite signals the need. Can you imagine how much life would be lost without it. It is a divine message from life to life.

If one looks at appetite with a recognition of its spiritual significance, one is moved to satisfy it in a way befitting its nature. Wholesome, tasty, natural foods, cooked to perfection in nature's wondrous variety is our heritage. Proteins are the building blocks of the body, fats and carbohydrates the fuel that activates it. Gastronomy is the study of preparing appetizing and nourishing food. It is a required course for the person who wants to stop interfering with his appetite through contrived diets. It provides ways to satisfy the taste senses while you satisfy body needs.

One wonders whether satisfaction is illegal or fattening, as the saying goes. More likely satisfaction is joy that nature means us to have when essential functions are carried out. It belongs with a sneeze, scratching an itch, performing the love act, or meeting hunger. Many of us have guilt feelings when satisfaction is enjoyed. Nature hints that it should be the other way around. We probably should feel guilty about pain, usually brought on by body abuse. We should exhult at the opportunity to satisfy bodily needs in a sensually gratifying way.

Appetite of any type, treated coarsely is bestiality. As advanced forms of life, we are capable of sensitivity and ingenuity. A marriage would soon flounder without these characteristics, as neither partner achieved self-realization. True fulfillment of the appetite for food also requires that sensitivity and ingenuity. With it, breakfast, lunch, or dinner becomes an event to be lived, not a job to be finished.

As you put the book down at the close of this chapter, stay a minute longer. Think about the long, long warehouses full of food for food's sake; of the millions of people who at this very moment are wolfing sandwiches or doughnuts just to fill their belly; and of the millions more whose ingenuity in titillating their taste buds begins and ends with sugar. Is there any wonder that their bodies fatten, and pains set in, as nature pleads stop!

10

How to
Stay Slender . . .

The time has now come when you can begin to visualize your-self slim. The last chapter in the fight against fat sees you as the victor in the fight against carbohydrates. You stop starvation dieting and you lose weight. Not only do you radiate new youth and exuberance, but you get more fun out of life, while you enjoy eating and drinking even more than you did in overweight days.

The best part of all is the peace of mind that comes with being off the diet treadmill. You now belong to the slender society, the people who can eat all they want and never be overweight.

. . . For Years

It has taken fattening carbohydrates a half century to engulf civilization. It has taken you just a few weeks to tear down old eating habits and build up new ones.

But civilization is not changed. You will be subjected to a constant carbohydrate barrage. Television commercials will show size 8 models drinking beer, munching candy bars and breakfasting on cereal. Your family, your associates and friends will offer you cake, potato chips, and pizza. Radio, magazines and billboards will bombard you with handsome and successful people eating 36 flavors of tangy ice cream, drinking any number of ice cold sodas and nibbling crackers, cookies and cakes. But you will know that all are exhorting you to buy yourself a fat profile; that in reality they are asking you to trade a day off your life in the future for a few minutes of saccharine pleasure now. It will not be likely that you will quickly slip off the bedrock of protein into that gooey carbohydrate mess. But this bombardment can gradually erode your new found protein habits unless you insulate yourself from its efforts.

When a doughnut shop recently tried heart-shaped holes they could hardly keep up with the demand, even at twice the price. There are now over 40 different types of doughnuts sold in shops across the country each competing with the next in eye appeal and doughnut sales are booming. You are not a regular customer today, if you have become a carbo-cal counter. But will you be tomorrow?

How To Keep From Changing Back

How do non-smokers resist the appeal of cigarette ads and commercials year after year, in fact permanently? Their greatest insulation from the strong motivations offered—fresh taste, a lift, relaxation—is the memory of a bad taste and the knowledge of the price to be paid for that lift or relaxation.

Similarly, a promise of carbohydrate pleasure will be recognized for the illusion that it is, if the memory is still fresh of the unwanted pounds, the tight clothes, the lagging health, and the looming shadow of age. You have been there. You know.

It is said that an alcoholic must hit bottom before he or she can expect to change. An over-weight person does not have to break the scale in order to effect a permanent break with the past, but somebody who has known the tortures of obesity and wins out over it the high protein way is less likely to succumb again quickly to the carbohydrate bombardment that the mere 15 or 20 pound loser. Both may sooner or later have to resort to a sort of reminder therapy, though, and here are some of the techniques that can be used.

First, and foremost; keep this book handy not only as a reference for carbohydrate value of foods, but as re-charge station. Find yourself eating a doughnut one day and that is the tip-off that it is time to re-read this book and remind yourself of the dangers of the carbohydrate morass.

Two; put up your own counter-barrage. Be a vocal proponent of nourishing, high protein foods. Remind others of the fattening nature of carbohydrate foods. Talk up a balanced, high protein fare and you re-enforce your own conviction.

Three; use the power of suggestion to nullify the effects of the carbohydrate bombardment. Tell yourself that what you are seeing or hearing is not good for you. Take your thoughts off the spaghetti and turn them on your favorite haute cuisine—cornish hen, shrimp creole or beef ragout.

One executive, who was a 235-pound spaghetti-lover, lost 20 pounds in six weeks just by substituting cheese for his daily spaghetti. Later, whenever the temptation to return to spaghetti became undeniable he would go to an Italian restaurant and order some flavorsome Roman or Venetian dish such as veal Parmesan, or Italian meat balls and tomato sauce. It turned the trick, as it was not the spaghetti he craved but the lusty flavors of the sauces that went on it—the taste of garlic, oregano, basil, etc.

There is hardly a craving that cannot be satisfied by a protein substitute and therefore no need to let a desire build up to a craving. Cream pies can be headed off by puddings with whipped cream. Pizza pies can find a reasonable facsimile in au gratin casseroles using similar topping ingredients.

Be A Protein Ambassador

To talk up high protein foods not only refreshes your protection against the carbohydrate barrage, but also helps to stem the growing tide of carbohydrate that is unbalancing the twentieth century diet. Bread and breadstuffs have turned from the staff of life to its crutch. As civilized man limps along the obese trail, up and down farinaceous mountains, skirting fat-connected diseases, on-and-off diets, the mountains grow higher, the diseases more prevalent and the diets less effective.

Public opinion can turn that tide. If the public wants a variety of easy-to-heat-and-eat meats, fish, eggs and cheeses, technology will find a way to produce them and capital will find a way to service that demand at a profit. Look at the tremendous industry that has been developed overnight in so-called non-fattening no-calorie foods. Canned fruits, fruit juices, soda lead an ever-increasing list of items now prepared with sugar substitutes that reduce calories to much lower levels. However, they are not the final answer. It does not serve the cause of longevity to wash down potato chips and pretzels with low calorie coke. Furthermore, the chemicals used in artificial sweeteners have not yet proved themselves to be harmless when used in volume or over an extended period of years.

The final answer is a new industry of prepared proteins that will gradually replace the carbohydrate era with a new age of ready to eat lobster Newburgh and beef bourguignon. New packaging coupled with new kitchen appliances—such as the infra-red oven—can bring the world of gourmet foods to the threshold of our present day demand for instant foods.

But first the present rise in weight consciousness must evolve into carbohydrate consciousness. Here is where you enter. Dieting is a bore. Anyone who has ever dieted will be anxious to hear about your experiences in staying slim. How do you do it? What about breakfasts? Don't you get hungry? Do you give up drinking? Aren't you hungry? These are the questions they will ask, and the answers you give will tell the story of carbohydrates. One more person will be alerted to the imbalance in our way of eating. If they comment that it sounds like a life-long diet, ask them if eating all you want for breakfast, lunch and dinner sounds like a diet. And ask them what diet they know of includes such gourmet specialties as grilled whole sea bass anbeurre, tongue mousse, lobster fra diavolo, veal picato, pot au feu, roast rack of lamb, steak bernaise, eggs benedict and banquets from turtle soup to strawberries and cream.

Intrigue them by name dropping. Like Kekoska U Umaku Od Slacice. Oh, didn't you know? That's Yugoslavian Chicken with Mustard Sauce. You roast the chicken. The sauce is made with the giblets, egg yolks, chicken stock, french mustard, wine vinegar, sour cream and a little rum. You pour the thickened sauce over the chicken, and it's divine!

If they challenge you on the dangers of high fat, rebut with the dangers of high *anything* including carbohydrates. Remind them that the body manufactures three times more cholesterol than they could ever eat. Tell them about the lean, sleek warriors called the Massi who live near Kenya, Africa, on a diet of something that contains enough cholesterol to send the worried American middle-ager fleeing from the table. These Africans live exclusively on meat, blood and milk with an average butterfat content of over 6%. Studies of the Masai show they have far lower serum cholesterol than the average American. And they have no hypertension in their keep-the-spears-sharp and watch-the-cattle society. Tell your dieting friends about the Eskimos, too, and their higher fat fare that produces no atherosclerosis. In between Africa and Alaska, you might infer, is a land where tension damages people and oftimes that damage is erroneously blamed on particular foods.

Go to work on teen-agers, especially. These adults of tomorrow are the sweet-snackers of today. They grow fat skipping breakfast, having a snack for lunch and eating junk for dinner if they can get away with it. In between are doughnuts, soft drinks, hamburgers, soft drinks, pizza slices, candy bars, potato chips, and more soft drinks. Talk them off the road to Fatsville and onto the nutritional protein-way. Let them eat from morning to night but let them eat right.

The Fork Can Be Man's Best Friend

Because time has allied itself with carbohydrates in this hurry-up age, the sandwich, the pizza slice and the cracker have zoomed in popularity. In effect, whenever time is saved for want of a fork, the cost is high in carbohydrates.

Take pizzas for example. They are now a serious challenge to the evening meal. It used to be a question of shall we have a frankfurter or a pizza, or a sandwich or a pizza. It is now shall we have dinner or a pizza. Pizzas have become a way of life. There is hardly a community without a pizza parlor.

Pizzas originated in Naples, Italy in the 17th Century. Common people ate folded pies in the streets. Later, society's upper crust took to it. However, it was basically a tomato pie until the 19th Century when mozzarella, a soft bland cheese, was added. Today toppings include, together or separately, Italian pork sausage, anchovies, spiced beef, garlic, onion, mushrooms, ham, salami, meat balls, green pepper. Some are even made with shrimp, tuna-fish, or mussels.

Do these toppings sound familiar? Yes, they are all high protein foods. Not a carbo-cal in a whole pie—except for that crust. In other words, if you had a fork, you could eat all the pizza you wanted providing you ate just the topping and left the pie shells. Don't be embarrassed, ask for a fork. And don't be ashamed to have a couple of extra slices.

A fork is a life-saver when it comes to sandwiches too. Most fast service lunch counters and restaurants serve a fork with the sandwich so that you can manage that side order of cole slaw or the tomato wedges. Take a few bites of the sandwich. What is a few carbo-cals among friends. But foil the armada of over 100 carbo-cals waiting to encircle you—at the waistline. Finish the sandwich, using the fork. Leave those few scraps of bread as a good-will offering, if your will is good enough.

At parties, instead of going for the canapes and instead of putting dips on chips or crackers, reach for a fork and a small plate. Help yourself to the chopped liver, the cheeses and the dips, taking small samples of each as you would with smorgasbord. Your fork can save you hundreds of unwanted carbo-cals and you can enjoy the party knowing that it has balanced the scales for you in favor of proteins.

The Price of a Carbohydrate Relapse

This may come as a surprise, but if you do succumb temporarily to the ingenious carbohydrate temptations that society can often devise, your lost week-end will not likely show at all on your scale in a few days. The reason is that a carbohydrate-heavy Saturday and Sunday is not likely to put more than a pound or two on you and that pound or two will be lost in the Monday through Thursday return to balanced eating at a 250 carbo-cal limit.

This is not to suggest that you go to carbohydrate hell with yourself on weekends and try to shape up in between. That would be defeating the whole non-diet, permanent weight control principle. Weekdays can be just as much of an eating and drinking binge as weekends if you do it right. By doing it right—the low carbohydrate way—you avoid slide-back Sundays and conscience-stricken Mondays.

But sometimes a week-end comes along where the party goer just cannot say no to the platters of sinful offerings that come along without breaking the festive spell. Or the food is so delicious that in satisfying your sensual delight, you over-satiate your appetite. These exceptions are insignificant in your total weight pictures and will continue to remain innocent enough as long as they remain exceptions and not the rule.

To insure that no tell-tale poundage remains to cause you penance, be especially careful of your carbo-cal intake for several days following a particularly rough week-end. Count every item looking it up in the table instead of resorting to memory. Size up your portions of carbo-cal content foods so that there is no chance to over-step the balanced 250-limit. In this way you reinforce your high protein ways so that they are not permanently swayed by the week-end revelry and at the same time prevent surplus carbohydrates to act as weight hooks to retain unwanted ounces.

There is no need to remind one of the fact that a more lengthy relapse can mean not only ugly poundage added to the body beautiful but the need to start from the beginning again in the retraining of the appestat and the re-educating of the palate. However, unless you are a very impressionable person, easily swayed by ads, displays, commercials and the person across the table from you, chances are there will be no such lengthy relapse. Actually there is no food that is denied you in the high protein fare. The limit of 250 carbohydrate calories per day always accommodate an occasional piece of cake or a Sunday malted, although there is no way to fit that in every day without seriously jolting your vitamin and mineral requirements.

Successful Defense Against the Carbohydrate Bombardment

One of the most effective defenses against the power of suggestions that urge you from all sides to sweets and starches is that very same power of suggestion—but used by *you* and *for* you.

The television screen can be just as powerful an aid to keep you on healthful, slenderizing protein as it is a tempter to sweets and starches. If you close your eyes and visualize a television screen, you can then turn on your own show. This is not a show where beer glasses clink and biscuits turn golden brown in the oven. This is instead a show where you are the star looking slender, youthful and vibrant. As you watch the show, you sit back comfortably in the chair. You are very relaxed. Nothing disturbs you. You can concentrate your full attention on the make-believe screen.

There you are now. Who is that you are with? You are dining on Steak Chateaubriand. You are having a good time. You look younger and radiate good health. The waiter is bringing the dessert now. It looks like a Casaba melon. Now the two of you are clicking your coffee cups together. As you leave, you notice how solid and trim of figure you are. You move with agility and seemingly without effort. You know that you have attained this state quite easily by eating the right foods—high protein "go" foods, and by avoiding high carbohydrate "stop" foods.

Men and women can elaborate on this imagining to their visual content, and each in their own way. It is a simple method of auto-suggestion that works in exactly the same way in your subconscious eating motivations as does the pretzel commercial or candy billboard. The deeper you are able to relax and the more vividly you are able to picture yourself, the sharper will the message be etched in the mind to protect you from ill effects any time that someone sings a song of sugar and starch.

The television screen method of auto-suggestion is also effective in breaking the back of a particular food habit that you find hard to get rid of. Suppose chocolate has steadily proven your downfall. You can aim some lethal suggestions at it that will sink it mighty fast. For instance, you can visualize a playlet where you are sitting in the living room. You see yourself go over to a bar of chocolate and take one. As you eat it, you fatten visibly. You take another and fatten still more. As you watch yourself eat the chocolate you can just feel how thick, bloated and distorted you must feel. Then you listen as you hear yourself say "Chocolate is on my stop list. It produces heavy, unwanted fat. From now on I will not desire chocolate. I will not even go near it. I will grow thin again on wholesome, nutritious foods. In fact, chocolate will no longer please my taste. It will give me no satisfaction. It will taste like the fat it becomes. I know now what damage it can do to my teeth, my health, and appearance."

The picture on your imaginary television screen then changes. You see yourself slender and attractive again. You are at a party. Someone offers you chocolate. You decline pleasantly. The end.

Instructions From Headquarters

The above television technique of auto-suggestion is used quite effectively in hypno-analysis and is in effect a type of mild self-hypnosis, just as commercials that appear on real television screens are a type of mild hypnosis. The sub-conscious is conditioned to obey instructions no matter from whence they come. That is why propaganda, even from a source that is recognizably hostile, can influence our beliefs. That is why, despite your protein resolve, carbohydrate contentment can be catching.

Every day people give themselves instructions that are implicitly obeyed. If we understood this and were more aware of it, we would hesitate at saying such things as so-and-so makes me sick, or, I just can't do that. We would be sure to give ourselves constructive and positive instructions that would expand our capability and improve our health.

Here are some of the positive suggestions that will help to keep knives, forks and spoons pointing due protein and away from excessive starches. You can make them to yourself via the television technique or merely by saying them out loud to yourself while seated in a comfortable chair and thoroughly relaxed:

I will not crave foods that are high in sugar and starch.

I will be satisfied with a normally moderate amount of food.

I will find meats, cheeses, fish, poultry, eggs thoroughly satisfying.

I will enjoy discovering new ways to prepare these nourishing foods.

I will find 250 carbo-cals sufficient for my needs.

I see myself staying permanently slim without dieting.

You will find it helpful to set a few minutes aside once a week for an auto-suggestion session, such as every Monday morning. It will reinforce the constructive steps you are taking to re-balance your diet the high protein way and insulate you against carbohydrate propaganda.

The instructions you give yourself will lessen the need for willpower. You automatically want to continue the high protein fun and your Stuffed Lobster or Veal Roulade and will never surrender to Fettucini Alfredo.

Picturing your auto-suggestions means visualizing yourself thin. Hold steadfastly to this picture. See yourself as you want to be, effervescing with bounce and vigor. Know that imagining furnishes the mind with a blueprint and this must come to pass if you see it so. Girls who have a dress in their closet that is impossibly tight can visualize themselves slipping into that very dress. Visualizing it can help to make it so, because your will is influenced by your mental picturing.

Sixteen Steps To Freedom From Diet

The steps outlined in this book are so simple that they should come naturally to everyone that tries them. But lest they have become buried in recipes, words and tables, let us outline them in simple step-by-step form to help you get started on the right foot and proceed successfully along the road to la dolce vita enjoyed by permanently slender people.

Step One   Assert your desire to be slim permanently. Forget all previous patterns of on and off dieting. Understand that by balancing your daily fare you can enjoy food and lose weight. Consult with your physician about your weight goals.

Step Two   Learn to recognize carbohydrates as the villain that unbalances modern eating. Memorize the food categories that are high in sugar, starch and other carbohydrates.

Step Three   Learn to recognize protein as the way to a balanced diet. Review your menus for meat, fish, poultry, cheese and egg dishes. They will replace menus with flour, potatoes and other high carbohydrate foods.

Step Four   Prepare a new shopping list shifting from high carbohydrate items to high protein items. Keep hands off the shelves you know to be dangerous.

Step Five   Make a typical 24-hour food intake analysis of your present diet. Record the time and portion of everything that goes into your mouth from chewing gum to beer.

Step Six   Place the carbohydrate value opposite every item on your intake analysis, using the table on page 110. Familiarize yourself with stop, caution and go foods in the table. Now add up your total carbo-cals.

Step Seven   Substitute high protein foods for high carbo-hydrate foods on your analysis table, starting with those with the largest carbo-cal content and working down the list until you have brought your total carbo-cals down to 250.

Step Eight   Prepare a number of typical menus based on your present eating habits—except protein foods are substituted for high carbohydrate foods. Retain a balanced amount of fruits and vegetables. Keep foods interesting and different.

Step Nine   Make food a hobby. Be adventureous. Learn new recipes. Try European and Oriental styles of cooking. Keep carbo-cals under 250, but eat all you want of "go" foods.

Step Ten   Prepare a progress chart. Plan to lose no more than 1% of your weight each week. Use "caution" foods as the adjuster, less when you want to lose faster, more when you stop losing.

Step Eleven   To maintain your weight, eat all you want of high protein foods. Don't deny yourself second portions or you may succumb to sweets later.

Step Twelve   Adopt the habit of daily exercise to tone up your muscles and firm up your figure. Don't expect to exercise weight off, just the wrinkles and the sag.

Step Thirteen   If your physician recommends a low fat diet for you, learn the difference between saturated and non-saturated fats and use the tables on page 214 to avoid foods with extra high fat content.

Step Fourteen   Screen the unwanted carbohydrates out of restaurant dishes and party snacks, using the hints in Chapter 8. Eat in fine places if you want, and enjoy the sensual pleasures of gourmet food. Partying can reduce obesity-causing tensions.

Step Fifteen   If your appetite sounds false alarms, retrain it according to the instructions in Chapter 9. Hold a mirror to your own personality traits to discover emotion-food relationships that you will want to correct.

Step Sixteen   Practice protein auto-suggestion to protect yourself from carbohydrate suggestions that surround you. Use imagining procedures in this chapter to solidify your new eating habits and speed the day when you attain your best weight and health.

These sixteen steps can be the greatest event of your life. What can you think of that is both fun and life-preserving? What else can ever get you off the diet treadmill and make you slim permanently?

The words *Youth, Vitality,* and *Health* have been used so frequently to describe the results of weight loss that they have little meaning in terms of tomorrow for the average person. Here is the way a 49-year-old salesman put it in his own words:

I know this sounds corny, but I am not the same person today that I was two months ago. I realize it every morning the second I open my eyes. I don't lie there in a stupor with a grey taste in my mouth. Instead I feel like bouncing out of bed right away.

When I dress and shave I am thinking about my activities for the day. I cannot remember feeling anything but ugly this early in the fat old days. But now if I could sing, I would. I have a good appetite. Instead of juice and coffee, I have a healthy order of bacon and fried eggs (over light).

I never realized that 25 pounds weighed so much. Without them, my step is jaunty and effortless. It makes me feel as if there is extra oxygen in the air. It is little wonder that my sales have gone up. My new enthusiasm seems catching. Sure, by 5 P.M. I start to fade. Then I enjoy a couple of Martinis and a good dinner and I'm back on top of the world. I can't say I feel younger; I know I'm not. But I know my insurance company has a better risk in me today than they had ten years ago.

These are not the words women use to describe the identical phenomenon. Their words are more likely to include "dresses fit," "men call," "feel better," "more energy," "greater confidence," and "cloud nine." Some say that when a man talks to them they are no longer self-conscious, that shopping is so much more fun, that they feel beautiful, and take better care of themselves.

The End Is The Beginning

Reindeer meat balls in gravy, mushrooms in brandy sauce, and salami studded gruyere cheese are some of the new gourmet foods—brimming with slenderizing protein—that have come on the American Market during the period that this book was being written.

There is a steady parade of products to delight the palate. All you have to do is tell the wheat from the chaff. We, the protein-conscious, discard the wheat and keep the chaff and stay thin. We would pass up the new Norwegian milk chocolate that melts in your hand as well as your mouth, we would want no part of the dried Mexican bananas, or the rum-flavored petit fours. Instead serve us a generous portion of that new escarole chicken broth, hot curry shrimp dip, or dried mango slices.

For we are the new breed of 20th century epicureans. Indulge us, if you please. We know how to eat and we know how to stop. We look back at those decadent decades of sweets and starches as days when we knew no better, days when our ignorance was paid for in pounds. We look ahead with a weightless wisdom to decades of protein promise. From martinis to whipped cream, bon appetit!

Index